Terpenes

The Magic Within Cannabis

Beverly A. Potter, Ph.D
"Docpotter"

with Abby Hauck

RONIN

Berkeley, California

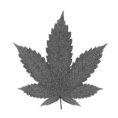

Important Notice:

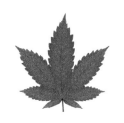

Terpenes

The Magic Within Cannabis

Beverly A. Potter, Ph.D
"Docpotter"

with Abby Hauck

Terpenes
The Magic Within Cannabis

Copyright 2019 by Beverly A. Potter
ISBN: 978-1-57951-272-9 Pbook
ISBN: 978-1-57951-273-6 Ebook

Published by

Ronin Publishing, Inc.

PO Box 3436
Oakland, CA 94609
www.roninpub.com

Production:
    Manuscript creaton: Beverly A. Potter.
    Cover Design: Brian Groppe.
    Book Design: Beverly A. Potter.
    Content Creation: Abby Hauck/CannabisContent.com
    Photos: Fotolia
Library of Congress Card Number: 2019931621

Distributed to the book trade by PGW/Ingram.

Acknowledgements

Thank you, Dear Reader, for picking up this book. May you find much to inspire you herein shared here in.

A special thanks to Abby Hauck for her assistance in the preparation of the manuscript.

—Docpotter

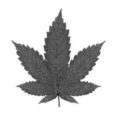

Table of Contents

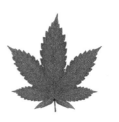

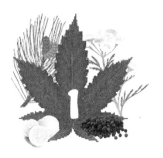

What Are Terpenes?

Commonly used in aromatherapy and religious practices, terpenes are the aromatic oils that give pine trees, soil, and yes, even cannabis, their unique scents and aromic appeal. Terpenes are fragrant molecules that occur naturally in many plants—especially conifers—and even in some insects. There are thousands of different terpenes, each with its own unique odor and flavor composition.

The word "terpene" is derived from the word "turpentine" because it is a major component of rosin and turpentine used as a solvent for paints, varnishes, and cleaners. Turpentine was traditionally used in Chinese medicine to relieve discomforts like tooth pain *Terpenes are the aromatic oils that gives cannabis strains their unique aromic appeal.* and breathing issues. Today it is more commonly used as a thinning agent for paints and varnishes thanks to its powerful solvent properties.

Turpentine

Most turpentine is made from coniferous trees—particularly pine and spruce—and is created one of three ways:

Gum Turpentine: The oldest procedure for making turpentine involved tapping trees to extract the sap (gum) then distilling the sap using steam to create turpentine.

Wood Turpentine: Wood turpentine is made with wood chips that are steam distilled to produce a turpentine oil.

Sulphate Turpentine: The most common turpentine extraction process used today, sulphate turpentine is a by-product of paper-making. Sulphate turpentine is collected from the gas that is produced during the pulping of wood and is often burned on-site as a power source for paper-making facilities.

Terpenes and Terpenoids

Terpenes encompasses a large group of unsaturated hydrocarbons that consist of at least one isoprene unit created by the formation of eight hydrocarbon and five carbon atoms—C_5H_8. Terpenes are classified according to how many isoprene units they composed of; monoterpenes consist of two isoprene units, diterpenes consist of four, triterpenes from six and so on. Though most cannabis-derived terpenes are classified as monoterpenes, some more complex—and less volatile—terpenes can be introduced into cannabis concentrates or otherwise consumed to improve flavor and act therapeutically on the body.

Though often used interchangeably, the terms "terpene" and "terpenoid" refer to slightly different chemical compounds. Basically, terpenes are the backbone, or the precursor, or terpenoids; they contain only their isoprene units—hydrogen and carbon—and nothing else. Terpenoids are terpenes that have been modified—either synthetically or organically—with heat, oxygen, or time. In terms of cannabis, this usually occurs during the curing process which immediately follows harvest.

Terpenes are also the precursor of steroids—like hormones—and other chemicals in the body. This explains their profound impact on the body, which will be discussed more in the coming pages.

Interest in terpenes has grown since cannabis legalization began. Between 2016 and 2018, internet searches for "terpene" jumped five percent thanks to its regular association with cannabinoids and other alternative medicines. What exactly are terpenes? Are they really as important as everyone seems to think?

Terpenes are extremely volatile and evaporate quickly at moderate temperatures—which is why morning air tends to smell "fresher" than evening air, because plant terpenes are at their peak of fragrance in the morning before the sun has come out to evaporate them. Cannabis cultivation and extraction experts often choose morning hours to harvest—and in some cases flash freeze—their crops at peak terpene levels.

Preserving terpenes after harvest is a delicate procedure and absolutely necessary if growers hope to capture the best flavor and scent of the cannabis plants while extending the shelf-life of the products. The process requires careful temperature and humidity control, or direct extraction from fresh or flash-frozen flowers. Terpene and terpenoid extraction will be discussed in further detail in a later chapter.

Discovery of Terpenes

Terpenes have been used for religious purposes dating back to Ancient Egypt. In 12th Century Europe, terpene extraction via lipids—oils and fats—was perfected with a focus on herbs like rosemary and sage. By 1589, more than 60 different essential oils were outlined in the book, *Dispensatorium Valerii Cordi* by Arnaud de Villanosa—up from only three just 44 years earlier—which highlights the interest and understanding of essential oils at the time. Pharmacists spent years perfecting the distillation process after noticing the profound effects these essential oils seemed to have on over-all health and well-being.

In 1818, the oldest known essential oil of turpentine was submitted for analysis where the isoprene molecule—C5H8—was first discovered. It was later discovered that all terpenes have this same ratio.

The term "terpene" was first coined in 1866 by scholar, Fr. A. Kekulé. His work opened the doors to a major discovery by Otto Wallach who noted a pattern of carbon to hydrogen atoms in all essential oils. Though the number of hydrogen and carbon atoms varied, the ratio was always the same: five carbon atoms to every eight hydrogen atoms. This introduction of the "isoprene rule" later earned Wallach a Nobel Peace Prize and landed him the title of "Messiah of Terpenes".

As more essential oils were discovered—and attention surrounding them grew, their applications expanded. Though their medical properties were still of interest, essential oils became more frequently used as perfumes and food additives. This expansion led to a boom in popularity now referred to as the "Elizabethan Age" of essential oils. Even today new essential oils are constantly being discovered followed by research into their composition, which helps researchers learn to isolate the aromatic compounds and synthesize them in laboratory settings.

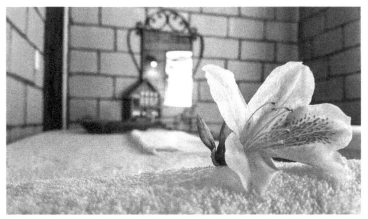

Oils used in aromatherapy are terpenes.

Therapeutic Benefits of Terpenes

Terpenes, or more specifically "aromatherapy" has been used for centuries for medical and spiritual purposes. While the term itself didn't originate until 1937, archaeological discoveries suggest that the use of medicinal herbs predates recorded history.

The use of aromatic plants in medicine dates back to 2800 BC in China. Texts outlining the power of plants, herbs, and spices included the stimulating effects of orange and the healing qualities of ginger. Later, in Ancient Egypt, the first collection of medical knowledge included the benefits of aromatic plants and their extracts on the body—both internally and externally—and on the mind. Plants were often burned as offerings to the gods and oil extractions were used to embalm their royalty.

Though aromatic herbs are well-known for their impact on the mind, much of this stems from the belief that it is the herbs various scents and not their chemical composition that exert the effects. Because the olfactory receptors are connected to emotion, it stands to reason that stimulation of these receptors would have an emotional impact on an individual.

However, it is believed that terpenes interact directly with brain cells to regulate their activity—including with cannabinoid receptors—the receptors that enable cannabinoids, like THC and CBD, to interact with the body. No wonder terpenes and cannabinoids seem to go so well together! In fact, it is the terpenes that give cannabis strains their unique scents and the terpenes that are responsible for the more intricate effects of a marijuana high. Terpenes and cannabinoids are produced in the same glands of the female cannabis plant—the "trichomes"—making the little crystals that coat cannabis buds all the more important and appealing.

Terpenes give cannabis strains their unique scents.

Looking Forward

Though their structure is simple, terpenes play a vital role in animal and environmental health. Terpenes are the backbone of all living things, contributing pigment and odor to biological or-

Though their structure is simple, terpenes play a vital role in animal and environmental health. ganisms. They also serve an important role in the regulation of vitamin degradation and the biosynthesis of hormones in the body.

In the following pages, the many ways terpenes interact with the body will be discussed in detail, both directly and through biosynthetic activity, then expand on the subject by analyzing the evolutionary benefit of such action.

The unique ways terpenes interact with the endocannabinoid system to accentuate the therapeutic potential of cannabinoids through the "entourage effect" is explored. We'll look at other sources of terpenes, both natural any synthetic, and discuss the most effective ways to collect and preserve these volatile—fragile—substances.

Finally, terpenes and flavonoids will be compared, to analyze the most common—and effective—ways to ingest them for therapeutic benefit, tips offered for cooking with terpenes, along with cautionary advice when dealing with these powerful—and sometimes toxic—compounds to ensure that everyone remains safe and healthy when using and ingesting terpenes into their daily regimen. So sit tight! Our adventure into the wonderful world of terpenes is just beginning.

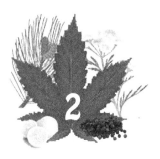

How Terpenes Work

Have you ever wondered why rainy days feel relaxing? Or why a day in the garden can be uplifting? A walk in the woods invigorating? Or why the smell of homemade apple pie makes think of Grandma? The answer: Terpenes.

Terpenes are aromatic oils that modulate mood and improve feelings of well-being, and not just because they smell good. Terpenes have incredible power over basic bodily functions. That they smell—and taste—good is a pleasant evolutionarily design enticing us to ingest them.

Terpenes modulate mood and improve feelings of well-being.

Terpenes and the Ecosystem

Humans, animals, insects, plants and fungi are part of a larger ecosystem sustaining life on this planet. In the grand scheme of things, we, too, are a part of Mother Earth. Terpenes play a vital role in maintaining homeostasis of our ecosystem.

Protection from Pests

Scientists believe that terpenes evolved to protect plants from pests by repelling them, by killing them, by trapping them in their sticky resin, and by attracting predators that eat them. Typically, terpenes work through unpleasant smells that deter pests, whereas pleasant smells attract beneficial insects and animals that prey on herbivorous insects eating them.

The glandular hairs of the plant is the main terpene production site and gives off a strong odor when their vapors are released. The pungent odor that the hairs give off can play a key role in protecting the plant from fungal infections, certain bacteria, and insects. Additionally, terpenes fragrances attract pollinating insects. Other terpenes have evolved a bitter taste that deters herbivores from eating them. Often terpenes are given off when the plant is stressed.

Terpenes promote life, protecting it from danger, and activating chemical reactions encouraging us to thrive at an optimum level. It should come as no surprise that terpenes—which are abundant in nature—can affect us more powerfully when we spend time surrounded by them.

Forest Bathing

A 2018 analysis of databases across the globe found that people who spent more time in green spaces as opposed to urban areas had lower levels of cortisol—the stress hormone—lower cholesterol, reduced risk of diabetes, and improved heart health. Pregnant women were less likely to give birth prematurely or to deliver underweight children. Overall, those who spent time in nature—no, looking out a window at some trees doesn't count—reported

The healing way of Shinrin-yoku Forest Therapy is simply being in the forest. Shinrin-yoku is a term that means "taking in the forest atmosphere—developed in Japan in the 1980s and has become a cornerstone of preventive health care and healing in Japanese medicine.

better health than those who didn't according to Twohig-Bennett and Jones' research. Some studies suggest a link between green space exposure and an improvement in cancer symptoms, neurological disorders, and sleep disturbances but research to support such claims is spotty at best.

Though there are many theories as to why people feel better after a day in nature—increased physical activity, sun exposure, and social interaction, for example—a more holistic factor may be at play. According to a 2009 study by Kobayashi's team published in the *International Journal of Immunopathology and Pharmacology*, phytoncides—organic compounds made from terpenes like pinene, cineole, camphene and limonene—

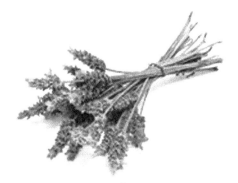

Linalool found in lavender, basil, coriander and citron is soothing.

decrease stress hormone levels in blood and urine analysis. They note that a "green prescription" may improve the effectiveness of medication in addition to its mental health benefits.

Considering the popularity of "forest bathing"—especially in Japan— Cho's research team analyzed a list of the most common terpenes found in Korean forestry like pinene, camphene, sabinene, camphor, limonene, cymene, menthol, and myrcene. They found these terpenes exerted many potential therapeutic benefits, the most common included anti-inflammatory benefits, anti-cancer properties, and neurological protection.

Anti-Inflammatory Effects

Pinene, a common terpene found in rosemary and coniferous trees, has been shown to reduce inflammation associated with bronchitis, ear edema—ear swelling, chronic obstructive pulmonary disease, osteoarthritis and skin inflammation. Pretreatment of rat models showed a marked decrease in allergic reactions, especially when used in conjunction with terpenes from frankincense, linalool and 1-octanol. Similar anti-inflammatory response have been found in human models, as well, suggesting that common terpenes could be an excellent tool through which to control chronic inflammatory diseases.

Limonene, another common terpene found primarily in citrus fruits, exerts anti-inflammatory properties likely due to its antioxidant qualities. It was shown to reduce cell migration—the birth and collection of new cells, cytokine production, and protein extravasation—all of which evoke inflammatory responses in the body.

Limonene found in citrus, works to protect against tumor growth.

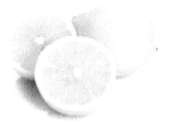

The monoterpene, p-cymene, showed promise as an anti-inflammatory agent and may, in fact, protect against future inflammation in the lungs such as that caused by cigarette smoke. Other terpenes with anti-inflammatory characteristics include linalool—found plants like lavender, basil and coriander, citron, and terpinene—found eucalyptus and cannabis.

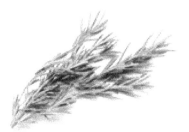

Pinene found in pine and rosemary, protects against tumors was signitificantly stronger in natural settings than in a laboratory.

Anti-Tumor Properties

Proliferation of tumors is multifaceted, including uncontrolled cell growth, weakened cell apoptosis, invasion activation and metastasis. Some terpenes have been shown to reduce tumor growth by acting on these pathways.

The most well-known terpene to exert anti-tumor properties is limonene, which is concentrated in the skin of many citrus fruits. It is powerfully effective in protecting against chemical-induced tumor growth including those that occur in the breasts, liver, pancreas, intestines and colon. Studies show that limonene stops tumor proliferation by inducing cell apoptosis and by suppressing the PI3K/Akt pathway, an intracellular pathway designed to regulate the cell cycle.

Pinene has been shown to protect against tumors by inducing G2/M cell cycle arrest, a process through which cells are instructed to attempt repair before producing new cells. It is important to note, however, that pinene exerts these qualities in natural settings significantly better than in a laboratory. Researchers observed better tumor control in mice that were kept in natural forested settings compared to lab rats, which suggests that pinene's positive effect may be due to a number of factors beyond simple administration.

Other terpenes that show promise in preventing and reducing tumors include perillyl alcohol—a metabolite of limonene, p-cymene, caryophyllene, and myrcene. These terpenes have demonstrated ability to attack solid tumors and prevent tumor growth while leaving surrounding cells virtually untouched suggesting that these terpenes could be used in conjunction with chemotherapy to improve its effectiveness.

Anti-inflammatory characteristics of borneol helps protect the brain from neurological damage.

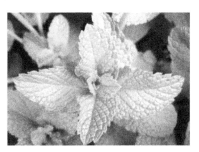

Neurological Health

While several terpenes are believed to have neurological benefits, supportive research has been limited. Only a few terpenes have been researched in regards to neuroprotective and regenerative properties. The most well-studied terpene in this category is called borneol derived from camphor trees.

Borneol contributes to neural health by acting as an antioxidant in the brain, sweeping up dan-

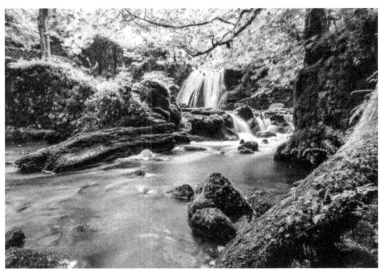

Inhaling a deep breath in a woodsy or forested area allows thousands of different terpenes to enter into the body to work their magic.

gerous free radicals in both in living and invitro—test tube—models. Anti-inflammatory characteristics of borneol helps protect the brain from neurological damage, suggesting that borneol may serve as a novel treatment in neurodegenerative diseases where oxidative stress is a major contributing factor. Synthetic forms of borneol show the similar therapeutic potential.

Other monoterpenes, like pinene and 8-cineole, exert neuroprotective properties by regulating gene expression. They protect cells from

Because they evaporate easily the best time to ingest natural terpenes is in the morning just before the sun comes out to burn them off.

apoptosis caused by oxidative stress and enhance the expression of antioxidant enzymes. More research is needed, however, to fully understand how these terpenes—and others—exert these beneficial qualities on the brain.

Terpene Absorption

The quickest and most effective method of terpene absorption is via inhalation, which explains why a breath of fresh air is so refreshing. Inhaling a deep breath in a woodsy or forested area allows thousands of different terpenes to enter into the body to work their magic. Terpene vapors can have an immediate impact on the body and mind—within seconds—affect our senses—they smell and taste amazing—as well as neurotransmission in the brain.

Terpenes are extremely volatile—they evaporate easily—which means that the best time to ingest natural terpenes is in the morning just before the sun comes out to burn them off. This explains why morning air seems to smell so much fresher than later in the day,

Terpenes protect the skin—and plants that create them—from dangerous ultra violet radiation—UV rays.

and is the reason most plants are harvested for their terpene content during the morning.

Topicals

Inhalation is not the only avenue through which terpenes get absorbed in the body. Topically-applied terpenes can penetrate the outermost layers of the skin—though only some have the capacity to break into the bloodstream through topical application. Interestingly, some terpenes actually improve the absorption rate of other topical medications, making them an excellent addition to topical creams and ointments.

A 2012 study published in the *Journal of Advanced Pharmaceutical Technology & Research* found nerolidol, from plants like jasmine, ginger, lavender and tea tree, to be the most effective in speeding topical absorption rate followed by farnesol, limonene, linalool, geraniol, carvone, fenchone, and menthol respectively. Dense terpene concentrations seem to work better than emulsified oils though some may cause irritation to the skin. It's important to understand the exact terpenes being used along with their toxicity levels when making homemade topicals and creams.

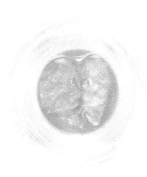

Terpene Sauve

Often, threats to plant survival come, not from a predator, but from a hostile environment. Extreme environmental conditions stress plants, threatening their survival. To combat this, some plants evolved a process to protect from extreme conditions by coating the plant's surface with reflective terpene oils. In other cases, plant terpenes evolved a way to release vapors into the atmosphere to shield it from harmful UV rays. The theory is that over millennia terpenes "learned" to create a kind of "cloud barrier" when exposed to high temperatures to increase air flow around the plant, reducing perspiration and limiting dehydration, as an example.

> *The theory is that over millennia terpenes "learned" to create a kind of "cloud barrier" when exposed to high temperatures to increase air flow around the plant.*

Terpenes protect the skin—and plants that create them—from dangerous ultra violet radiation—UV rays. Of particular interest are terpenes like limonene—citrus, which protect the skin from irritation and cymene—eucalyptus, which encourages new skin growth.

Labuda and Burns' research showed that terpenes protect the skin—and plants that create them—from dangerous ultra violet radiation—UV rays. Of particular interest are terpenes like limonene—citrus, which protect the skin from irritation and cymene—eucalyptus, which encourages new skin growth. They filed a patent application for their methds of using terpenes and terpenoids to block ultraviolet radiation and promote skin growth.

Of course, the use of terpenes in topical creams is not new—people have been using terpene-infused anti-aging creams to reduce wrinkles and aloe-based lotions to calm sun burns for centuries. Our better understanding of terpenes and their effect on the body helps to understand how these products are so popular—and effective.

Terpenes are all around us and contribute to well-being in numerous ways. They help us live our best, healthiest lives by improving physical and mental health. But terpenes have played a much more intricate role in our evolution than simply making us feel good.

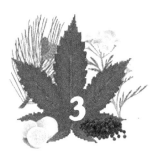

Types of Terpenes

Terpenes are responsible for many of the physiological and psychoactive effects that cannabis is known for. Following are some of the major terpene isolates found in cannabis along with associated "entourage effect."

Limonene

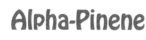

Limonene (lim o kneen) is a major terpene responsible for both flavor and effects in sativa cannabis strains. Found in other sources, such as citrus fruits, this terpene aids in the absorption of other terpenes through the mucous membranes and epidermis. In concentrated form, limonene is used to help with both anxiety and depression.

Alpha-Pinene

A-pinene (alpha pine knee nnn) is found naturally in

pine trees, turpentine and other coniferous plants. A-pinene is an abundant variety and is responsible for much of the odor associated with cannabis strains. It acts as an anti-inflammatory agent and bronchodilator.

Linalool

Linalool (lin a lool) is noted for its floral scent that is similar to spring flowers and is one of the more interesting terpenes found in cannabis. Linalool is popular for its sedative properties and ability to act as an effective anxiety and stress reliever. Linalool has both analgesic—pain relief and antiepileptic properties.

Myrcene

Myrcene (meer seen) is the most prevalent of all terpenes found in cannabis. Interestingly, the concentration of myrcene in a cannabis plant determines whether that strain is considered an indica or sativa. Cannabis strains that contain a myrcene concentration of 0.5 percent or less produce an energizing effect, while strains containing over 0.5 percent produce a more sedative effect. Myrcene is also found in hops, lemongrass, citrus fruits and thyme and is often used in aromatherapy.

Terpinolene

When inhaled, terpinolene (ter pin o lean) produces a sedative effect, according to researchers Ito and Ito. Terpinolene has been shown to exhibit potential anticancer and antioxidant effects, leading some researchers to believe that terpinolene will become a valuable medicinal tool.

Geraniol

Found in geraniums, geraniol (ger ayn e ol) gives off a rosy scent making it a popular extract used in perfumes. Geraniol can repel mosquitos and presents a potentially protective effect against neuropathy, a type of degenerative disease that affects the nerves outside of the brain and spinal cord.

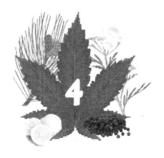

The Entourage Effect

Israeli chemist Raphael Mechoulam isolated THC in 1964 in collaboration with Dr. Yechiel Gaoni and Dr. Yuval Shvo. The discovery of Tetrahydrocannabinol (THC)—a primary cannabinoid—marked the beginning of medicinal marijuana research. In 1988, it was discovered that cannabinoids interact with special "receptor cells" found throughout the body to provide therapeutic results. They named it the "Endocannabinoid System" (ECS).

As breeders learned about cannabinoids and their impact upon the ECS, they set out to increase the concentration of cannabinoids in their plants. Strains have been selectively bred to be more potent, extraction methods perfected to reduce the plant matter in smoked marijuana, and distributors upsell the cannabinoid profile to consumers.

This is just the beginning of discoveries about medicinal cannabis. Research has revealed that cannabinoids are not the only chemicals that interact with cannabinoid

Terpenes are hydrocarbons—compounds of hydrogen and carbon—called isoprene molecules. Each isoprene molecule contains five carbon atoms with double bonds. The simplest terpenes are monoterpenes that contain two isoprene molecules. Sesquiterpenes have three isoprene molecules and and **diterpenes** *have four.*

receptors—there are other powerful chemicals in cannabis flowers called terpenes, the oils that give plants flavour and smell, can have powerful therapeutic benefits.

Swiss scientist, Jürg Gertsch and his colleagues in 2008 discovered that beta-caryophyllene—a sesquiterpene found in black pepper, oregano, cannabis and other leafy vegetables—interacts with CB2 receptors in the ECS, which are found in the body's peripheral tissue—skin, stomach, lungs; but not the brain or spinal cord. Beta-caryophyllene is considered both a terpene and a cannabinoid and is commonly referred to as a "dietary cannabinoid".

Since Gertsch's discovery, other terpenes have been shown to interact with cannabinoid receptors. For example, when consumed alone THC

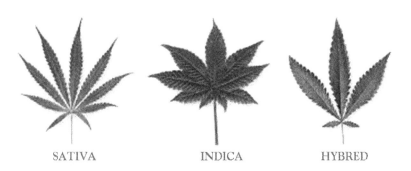

SATIVA   INDICA   HYBRED

may cause a reduced perception of pain, the intricacies of the "high", however, comes from the various terpenes in the cannabis. This is how some cannabis strains make us feel sociable, while others make us want to nap. It is the profile of the terpenes in the smoke, not the THC levels, that do it.

Lemon Skunk, for example, is a well-known sativa strain with a strong lemon-like flavor and a skunk-like undertone. Lemon Skunk is popular for its predictable effects: an up-beat sociable high perfect for busting the blues that helps us to come out of a gloomy shell.

The three types of cannabis plants are **indica** *and* **sativa** *and* **hybrid.** *Each strain has it's own range of effects on the body and mind resulting in a wide range of medicinal benefits.* **Indica** *strains provide a sense of deep body relaxation;* **sativa** *strains tend provide an energizing experience, with hybrids providing a cerebral high while relaxing the body.*

White Rhino, by comparison is an indica strain with a cannabinoid profile similar to that of Lemon Skunk. However, unlike Lemon Skunk, it delivers a slow but steady state of sedation, so that the effects of White Rhino are more calming and helpful in bringing on sleep.

If the cannabinoid profiles of Lemon Skunk and White Rhino are similar, what makes their effects so different? Is the answer that Lemon Skunk is a sativa-type strain, while White Rhino is an indica? That simple answer is correct, but the more complex answer is found in the effect of terpenes. While terpenes determine the flavor and aroma profile of the cannabis strain, they also determine the characteristics of the "high" as well.

For example, most citrus-flavored cannabis strains fall on the sativa side of the spectrum to promote activity, creativity and conversation; whereas musky flavored strains tend to be Indica and promote sedation. Further, while many factors, such as grow patterns and leaf structure, determine if a strain is sativa, indica, or hybrid, what is not well-known is that it is the terpene profile that determines when a strain will elevate or sedate our mood.

Interestingly, most indica plants tend to be smaller with a shorter phototropic period, tend to produce sedative terpenes while sativa plants that grow larger and take longer to flower, tend to produce uplifting terpenes. Building on this knowledge, breeders customized strains through multiple generations of selective cross-breeding.

The Entourage Effect

Dr. Ethan B. Russo published a break-through article in 2011 wherein he outlined the symbiotic relationship between cannabinoids and terpenes—both of which are produced in the trichomes of the cannabis flower. Trichomes are small oil–filled crystles that coat cannabis flowers. Cannabinoids and trichomes both begin as geranyl pyrophosphate that are then transformed into a terpenes or phytocannabinoid acids such as pentyl or propyl cannabinoid acid.

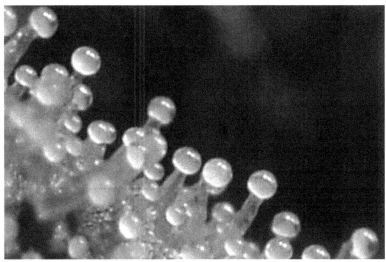

Trichomes are small oil–filled crystles that coat cannabis flowers.

Research has established that cannabinoids and terpenes come from the same chemical parent. Building on that, exciting research revealed that cannabis' effects go hand-in-hand with terpenes. Looking at past research on the subject, Russo compiled a list of studies to support the theory that full cannabis extracts—not isolated cannabinoids—provide stronger therapeutic benefit. Several studies—some from as early as the 1980s—have shown that terpenes work together to help cannabinoids—like THC and CBD—pass through the bloodstream easier and lower the blood-to-brain barrier. Naming the phenomena, "The Entourage Effect", Russo hypothesized that terpenes help modulate the effects of cannabinoids, which improves therapeutic effects

Simply stated, we feel more or less of the effects of a cannabis strain based on the terpenes found in it. The presence of small amounts of terpenes can boost therapeutic benefits of cannabis. According to the *Handbook of Essential Oils*, terpenoid concentrations above .05 percent are considered pharmacologically relevant because above this level there are significant physiological changes in the body. Mice exposed to terpenes, like linalool and pinene, in ambient air for one hour at a time demonstrated profound alterations in energy levels—even at low terpene concentrations. Terpene levels in mice were comparable to the pain-relieving THC levels in humans suggest-

The entourage effect refers to the way the different chemicals in cannabis work together, play off each other, and enhance or downplay the end effects. ing that both cannabinoids and non-cannabinoid terpenes can be therapeutically beneficial.

Terpenes have their own medicinal effects—apart from providing the tastes and smells of cannabis, they work together to amp up or chill out the dominant effects of the other cannabinoids. This is called the entourage effect because of the way the different components can work together, play off each other, and enhance or downplay the end effects.

How Terpenes Work

Terpenes have their own effects apart from their relationship with cannabinoids, including inhibiting serotonin uptake and enhancing norepinephrine activity—acting as antidepressants, increasing dopamine—regulating emotions and pleasure experiences, and augmenting GABA—the "downer" neurotransmitter associated with relaxing effects.

More research needs to be done about the compounded therapeutic effect of terpenes with cannabinoids on the mind, emotions, and behavior of consumers.

Currently, the accepted knowledge is that terpenes compound or lighten the effects of cannabinoids THC and CBD—among others—by binding to endocannabinoid receptors and neurotransmitters and imitating compounds our bodies naturally produce to regulate emotions, weight, health and well-being. The FDA and other agencies have recognized terpenes as safe, but how could they not? They'd have to outlaw tomatoes and cinnamon if terpenes weren't legal.

With research, cannabis scientists, growers, and enthusiasts are starting to tailor strains to use terpenes to balance the negative effects of cannabinoids—such as pinene balancing the short-term memory loss from high concentrations of THC.

The Sum of its Parts

A FDA-approved synthetic form of THC, called marinol, has been available to the public since the 1980's. Due to complaints about anxiety and confusion, however, its use is often discontinued, while using medicinal marijuana remains a popular choice for many Americans. It may be that marinol's lack of appeal is because it is THC only, without any other cannabinoids.

Terpenes have certain predictable effects on the body—such as pinene improves focus and linalool promotes relaxation. Though research is slim due to federal restrictions and unnecessary red tape regarding the cannabis research process, patients, breeders, and researchers alike agree that the interaction between terpenes and cannabinoids within the body can alter the effects of the high and contribute to the therapeutic potential of cannabinoids like THC and CBD.

There are hundreds of combinations of terpenes and cannabinoids that can be used therapeutically. Though individual results always vary, some basic combinations of cannabinoids and terpenes along with their therapeutic benefit are listed from the *Alchimia Blog*:

- *Pinene, linalool, and limonene:* This combination boosts the effectiveness of THC as well as working wonders on acne-prone skin, making it especially appealing for topical use.

- *Pinene, myrcene, and caryophyllene:* This powerful combination may be helpful in the treatment of addiction.

- *Limonene and linalool:* The fresh scent of these two terpenes help enhance the effects of CBD in the body.

- *Myrcene, linalool, and caryophyllene:* Combining these terpenes with THC helps to reduce anxiety and to promote sleep—making it a great combination for the treatment of sleep disorders.

Though there is still debate as to which is better, whole-plant cannabis extracts or cannabinoid isolates where terpenes—natural or synthetic—have been reintroduced, the fact remains that terpenes are an important part of cannabis therapeutics. Ignoring them means neglecting their importance to our overall health and turning our backs on years of research into the benefits of terpenes and their interaction with the body.

Flavonoids vs. Terpenes

Flavonoids sound like flavors… but they're actually the *color-giving* nutrients in living things. They're also one of the largest nutrient families known to scientists at over 6,000 members.

Around 20 of these compounds have been identified in the cannabis plant, which is great because they're also known for their antioxidant and anti-inflammatory health benefits.

Flavonoids are what gives cannabis plants a purple or brighter green color. Further research is needed to understand the role flavonoids can play for therapeutic cannabis treatments, but the research on terpenes is much further along.

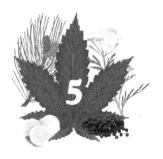

Natural Terpene Sources

Terpenes are among the oldest and most abundant biomolecules on the planet. There are thousands of known terpenes with new ones still being discovered. And though cannabis does produce a number of terpenes that vary by the strain, there are many other natural sources of terpenes that are also therapeutic.

Sources of Monoterpenes

Monoterpenes are the most volatile of the terpenes and the most abundant in nature. Monoterpenes emit unique fragrances as they evaporate, filling the air with perfumes. Monoterpenes are also the most common type of terpene found in cannabis, which includes limonene, pinene and myrcene among other terpenes.

There are, however, many other sources of natural monoterpenes that can be extracted to be used in conjunction with cannabis to boost the therapeutic potential of both.

Pinene is commonly found in cannabis and in conifer—evergreen—trees. Pinene is also found in some varieties of lime, in eucalyptus and in herbs like basil and rosemary. Though there are two different types of pinene—alpha-pinene and beta-pinene, they both offer the same therapeutic benefit. The major difference between the two is their aromas. A-pinene encompasses the smell of pine and rosemary, whereas b-pinene carries the scent of dill, parsley or basil.

Limonene, another monoterpene found in cannabis, is also found in citrus fruits like oranges and lemons—particularly concentrated in the rinds—

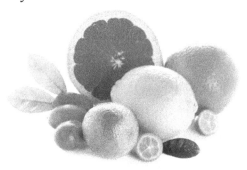

Terpenes are responsible for the characteristic aroma of many citrus fruits.

as well as in dill, fennel, celery and caraway seeds. The primary mode of limonene consumption is through food and beverage, however limonene is also readily released by plants into the atmosphere with concentrations varying by location. An orange grove in Southern California, for example, will have more limonene in the air than that in a city like New York.

Linalool is a popular floral-scented terpene abundant in many cannabis strains as well as in plants like cinnamon, rosewood, and birch trees. Though linalool is common in perfumes and other fragrances, one of its most common uses is as an antifungal and pesticide. Hence, linalool is an especially attractive ingredient in topical creams, flea baths, and bug repellants. Studies suggest linalool repels mosquitos up to 96 percent better than do citronella candles.

Myrcene is a musky, earthy terpene that tends to encourage sleep. Myrcene is the most prominent terpene in cannabis and is also found in significant concentrations in mangos, lemongrass, basil and hops—beer enthusiasts take note.

Myrcene increases penetration of the blood/brain barrier, making it an excellent addition to topical creams and ointments because they act as carrier agent through the skin into the bloodstream. Interestingly, myrcene consumed from food stuff, like mangos,

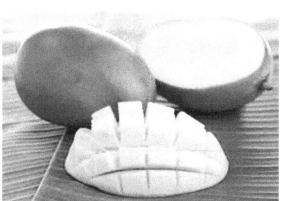

Myrcene is a musky, earthy terpene in mangos.

for example, can speed and intensify a marijuana high by giving THC and other cannabinoids a fast pass through the bloodstream and into the endocannabinoid system. In other words, the rumor that eating mangos before you get high will get you "higher" has substantial basis.

Myrcene's ability to penetrate the blood/brain barrier may explain why mixing beer and smoked cannabis can result in a case of the "spins". The myrcene from the beer's hops increases THC levels in the body while a drunk brain may commonly insist you aren't high enough. Though its also important to note that the consumption of any alcohol—regardless of the presence of myrcene—increases THC concentrations in the blood.

Sources of Sesquiterpenes

Sesquiterpenes occur in lower concentrations in cannabis but serve an important purpose. They are larger and more stable and tend to have a thicker consistency than monoterpenes making them especially prominent in concentrated forms of cannabis—as opposed to monoterpenes that often evaporate during the purging process—as well as in home-made edibles.

Finola was analyzed 2017 by Canadian researchers Booth, Page, and Bohlmann. A hemp cannabis strain, they determined the concentrations of the various terpenes found in the resinous glands of the cannabis flower. The team found many of the most common mono-terpenes—including pinene, limonene, and myrcene—as well as four sesquiterpenes

Caryophyllene is the most common sesquiter-pene found in the Canadian researchers' cannabis sample, with a concentration ranging from 13 to 46 percent. Caryophyllene is the only known terpene to interact with cannabinoid receptors to help enhance its pain-relieving and anti-inflammatory properties. There are large concentrations of caryophyllene in cloves—especially the stems and flowers, in rosemary and hops. In fact, though its concentrations are high in cannabis, caryophyllene can be extracted from a number of other sources including black pepper, basil, oregano, black caraway and, ylang-ylang.

Humulene is the second most prominent ses-quiterpene the Canadian researchers found in their cannabis sample with a concentration of up to 19 percent. Humulene shows exceptional anti-inflammatory properties and can be found in plants like ginseng, tobacco and sunflowers.

Farnesene, which is actually a precursor to humulene, that is, farnesene transforms into humulene through biosynthesis. Farnesene is commonly found in the skin of green apples—hence the sour flavor of Granny Smiths—and reacts strongly to oxidation that causes a damage in fruit. Therapeutically speaking, farnesene shows promise as an anti-inflammatory agent and may reduce the spreading of tumor cells. Most commonly found in indica-type cannabis strains, farnesene may be used to reduce muscle spasms. Other sources of farnesene include turmeric and sugarcane and in shark and olive oils.

Bergamontene is a sesquiterpene often used to treat stress, indigestion, infection, insomnia and inflammation. Concentrations of bergamontene were significantly lower than the other detectable terpenes at three percent on average, but still noteworthy. In addition to being found in cannabis, bergamontene can be extracted from carrots and tobacco and thought to be one of the plant's primary defenses against parasitic infestation. As such, it is often used to treat infections—especially those that produce excessive mucus—in addition to its anti-inflammatory properties.

Bacteria As a Terpene Precursor

Terpenes are well-known in various plants and fungi, but studies suggests that their formation may be born from bacteria. Japanese Yamada Research team from Brown University discovered that bacteria have an amazing genetic capacity to create terpenes. Prior to their study, there were 140 probable sequences for terpene synthesis, but the recent realization that bacteria synthesize ter-

penes bumped that number up to 262. By manip-
ulating just 13 of these newly discovered sequences, researchers were able to genetically engineer
completely new terpenes suggesting that there
are many more to be discovered.

The role bacteria play in the production of
terpenes is unclear, it may explain why microbes
often appear in cannabis lab tests. Though cannabis testing facilities must fail a product that tests
positive for microbial contamination, scientist
McKernan says that doing so may greatly limit
the concentration of beneficial terpenes.

There are many natural sources of terpenes
well beyond those found in cannabis. Even some
of the same terpenes found in cannabis can be
found elsewhere in nature then reintroduced into
cannabis products—food, drink, topical creams to
increase their therapeutic potential.

That plants, insects and animals use terpenes
to communicate gives much to muse upon. The
discovery that microorganisms use terpenes
to influence their world has huge implications
regarding the importance of terpenes in the environment. Indeed, all species have different
communication patterns, but terpenes seem to be
universally mis-understood. This "multilingual"
function of terpenes further highlights their evolutionary benefit as they are one of the few substances recognized by nearly every living thing
on the planet.

Cannabis Concentrates

Cannabis concentrates are substances in which excess plant matter has been removed to yield a concentrated form of highly potent tetrahydrocannabinol (THC) extraction that looks like honey or butter, which is why it is often called "honey oil" or "budder". Concentrates come in many different forms, including hashish, rosin, bubble hash, budder, shatter, and crumble. They can appear as a thick butter-looking substance, as a dark hard brick, in powder form, as an oil that varies in color, as a waxy residue, and even hard with the translucency of glass.

Concentrates may be called marijuana concentrate, extract, shatter, wax, butane hash oil or butane honey oil (BHO), live resin, budder, and taffy. Cannabis concentrates are available in many forms such as oils, wax, glass, shatter, and oral tinctures and obtained through an extraction process.

Concentrate

Growing Popularity

Popularity of concentrates is growing rapidly because they are much more potent than flower, thereby providing a more economical way to consume cannabis. The high potency may allow medicinal users to achieve faster relief than when smoking the flower or eating edibles.

The difference in flavor between concentrates and flower can be dramatic. Cannabis extracts not only concentrate cannabinoids, but the taste and beneficial terpenes are also concentrated. The flavor resulting from concentrate vaporization enables users to taste terpenes more clearly, instead of having the terpene flavor mixed with the taste of the combustible plant matter—as occurs while smoking flower.

Extracting Concentrates

Both cannabinoids and terpenes develop in the same part of the cannabis plant: the trichomes— the tiny mushroom-like crystals that form throughout the surface of the cannabis flower. The milky white trichomes resemble sand which makes the cannabis flower appear to have been dusted with the fine, potent powder. These trichomes are the same sandy substance that falls off freshly ground cannabis flowers, the same stuff that sticks to fingers after being handled and are the basis for all cannabis concentrates. In fact, one of the oldest forms of cannabis concentrates, hash, is made by collecting powdery trichomes then forming it into little balls. "Scissor hash" is simply trichomes that have been scrapped off trimming scissors.

The oldest method of creating concentrates involves crushing dried cannabis flowers with your hands or rubbing it through a screen—a process called "dry sifting", then wiping up the trichomes sticking to your fingers or the screen, and forming it into little balls of a dark amalgamation. The extracted powdery-appearing substance is commonly known as kief. Often heat and compression is used to convert the kief into blocks of hashish.

After extraction, the cannabis concentrate that remains has very high levels of terpenes and cannabinoids, especially THC, which can reach 80% or greater. Many extraction processes and specific strains of cannabis focus on extracting and creating high levels of medicinally beneficial cannabidiol (CBD) as high as 4%, which is considered exceptionally high.

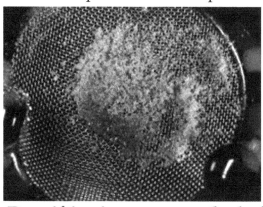

Dry sifting is an easy method of extracting kief from flower.

Extracting Without Solvents

Two modern extraction methods for creating cannabis concentrates are solvent-based extraction and non-solvent extraction. Gathering the trichomes on a screen, a trimming scissor, or on your hands are examples of non-solvent extraction because no solvent is used to gather or extract the sticky trichomes from the flower.

Kief

Kief is the simplest type of cannabis concentrate and comes from simply rubbing dried cannabis flowers on fine screens then collecting the sandy stuff that falls from them. Many cannabis-specific herbal grinders come with a special compartment designed for collecting keif that consumers may use to "top a bowl" of flower being smoked in a pipe. Sometimes kief is added to a marijuana cigarette or

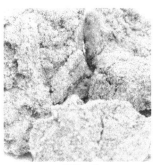

"joint" to improve its flavor and potency. Because there is no heat, pressure, or solvents needed to extract kief, the terpene profile of this type of cannabis concentrate matches the flower from which it came.

Kief

Hash

Hash is kief that's been shaped into a ball, cube, or chunk. Often it is made by rolling kief between the palms of the hand, which is then sliced and smoked by itself or added to cannabis flower and smoked.

Hash is one of the oldest forms of cannabis concentrate and was especially popular in Eastern Asia and the Middle East. Traditionally, hash has been exported for sale on the black market because it is easily condensed and transported.

Dry Sift

Dry sift is much like hash or kief except that it's been refined using a series of specially designed screens. Each screen has a different micron unit— different hole size—to separate plant matter from trichomes, separate large trichomes from small ones, and whole trichomes from broken ones. Only whole, plump trichomes contain the full terpene and cannabinoid profile of the flower.

Bubble Hash

Bubble hash gets its name from its extraction method, which involves agitating dried cannabis flower in ice

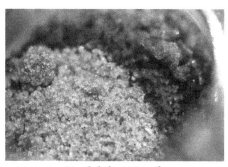

Bubble Hash

cold water to help frozen trichomes to fall off and collect in the bottom of a bucket. As the cannabis flower gets agitated, little air bubbles surface giving the mixture a fizzy, bubbly appearance. Bubble hash is a more thorough way to remove trichomes from cannabis flower as opposed to traditional hash extraction methods because it literally washes the trichomes from the plant, which are then collected in special mesh bags.

The quality of bubble hash depends on the size of the mesh screens, which range from 160 microns—large mesh holes—to 45 microns—very small mesh holes. Anything larger than 160 microns usually contains debris like dirt and unwanted plant matter, whereas micron levels lower than 45 tend to collect only damaged trichomes and fewer terpenes. Often, bubble hash producers use multiple mesh bags at once by stacking special micron bags by their size and then sell the resulting "bubble hash" based on the bag from which it was collected.

Full Melt Bubble Hash

Full melt bubble hash—Full Melt—is made using the same ice water bath as described for bubble hash with a few additional steps. First and foremost, full melt is made from freshly harvested cannabis that has been flash-frozen to preserve its cannabinoid and terpene profiles. Whereas cannabinoids and terpenes can break down or degrade over time, full melt omits the drying and curing—and thus the degradation—process to produce hash that is both potent and flavorful. Full melt will bubble and burn off completely when exposed to heat as opposed to regular bubble hash which may leave ash and other residue behind.

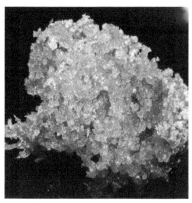

Full Melt Bubble Hash

Full melt is more refined than traditional bubble hash—and thus more expensive—but can be used in vaporizer pens as well as special oil pipes called "dab rigs". Traditional bubble hash, by comparison, should only be consumed in a pipe or a joint—but not in a vape or dab rig, or added to edibles.

Rosin

Rosin is the only non-solvent cannabis concentrate that resembles solvent-based concentrates. It is made by heating and pressing the resinous trichomes out of the plant and onto parchment paper. The sticky extract is then smoked in a pipe, in an oil (dab) rig or added to cannabis-infused edibles.

Distillates

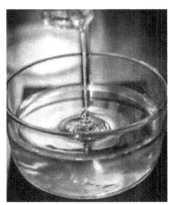

Distillate

Distillates are a newer form of cannabis concentrates and quickly becoming a favorite due to their extremely high potency with a lack of solvents. The distillation process uses heat and pressure to extract cannabinoids and terpenes by vaporizing them at specific temperatures. As the flower gets heated to the different temperatures, various substances get burned off or collected in tubes and saved for later.

Because terpenes evaporate quickly at low temperatures traditional distillation methods tended to yield lackluster cannabis concentrates. Emerging modern cannabis distillation methods trap the terpenes before they burn off for reintroduction into the cannabis concentrate later. Other natural terpenes—those that are not extracted from the cannabis plant—may also be added to distilled cannabis concentrates.

Extracting With Solvents

Solvent-based extraction involves using a liquid to remove the trichomes from the plant matter by dissolving them in a solution. When extracting with a solvent, hydrocarbons like butane, CO_2, ethanol, hexane, or propane are used to separate out the psychoactive compound THC, other cannabinoids and terpenes from the plant matter.

Increasingly concentrates are being made using different types of solvents to help strip cannabinoids and terpenes from plant matter into alcohols, fats and gaseous materials. Below are common types of solvent-based cannabinoid extraction methods.

Butane Hash Oil

Butane is one of the oldest solvents used for cannabinoid extraction. Butane hash oil (BHO) is made by placing marijuana flower or trimmings into a special tube, which is then filled with butane to strip the cannabinoids and trichomes from the plant. Next the butane is squeezed

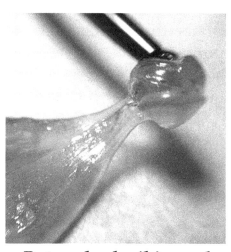

Butane hash oil is good for dabbing

from the tube while the plant matter stays behind. The gaseous material is then removed or purged leaving only cannabinoids and terpenes. The final result can take many forms that resemble things like butter—"budder", honeycomb, which is often dry, crumbly, and porous, wax, which is often soft like ear wax, or shatter, which is an amber-colored substance that looks like hard candy.

Unfortunately, many terpenes are lost during the butane purging process because of their volatile nature. Some companies rectify this issue by reintroducing terpenes into their cannabis concentrates.

CO_2 Oil

CO_2 is the same stuff that adds carbonation to soda, which makes it safer to consume than BHO—though note that, if BHO is thoroughly purged, it is considered safe to consume. CO_2 also helps keep terpene profiles in tact resulting in a more flavorful cannabis concentrate.

CO_2 extraction utilizes heat and pressure to remove both cannabinoids and terpenes from the cannabis plant. Extractors can adjust heat and pressure to optimize the extraction process while maintaining the quali-

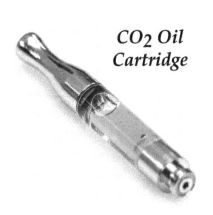

CO_2 Oil Cartridge

ty of the terpenes and cannabinoids via a process called "supercritical CO_2 extraction". This allows extraction technicians to harvest terpenes from the cannabis plant in a separate receptacle for re-

introduction into the
cannabis concentrate
later in the process.

Live Resin

Much like the full
melt bubble hash, live
resin is made by first
flash freezing can-
nabis flowers to pre-
serve the terpene and
cannabinoid profiles.

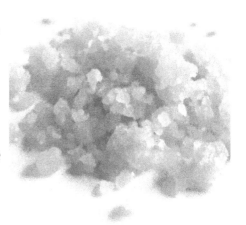

Live Resin

In fact, any cannabis concentrates that are labeled
with the term "live" means they have been flash frozen prior to the extraction process for a more flavorful, more potent concentrate.

Live resin is made in the same way as BHO—
plus the extra freezing process—resulting in concentrates like live resin—much like the shatter
or the candy-like concentrate mentioned earlier,
live sugar—a crumbly, sugary substance, and live
budder, which features a smoother texture and
easy malleability.

Tinctures

Cannabinoids are easily absorbed into alcohol
making alcohol a great solvent for cannabinoid
extraction. Tinctures are one of the easiest cannabis concentrates to make, requiring only a little
weed and high proof alcohol to leach the canna-

binoids out of the plant. After the cannabinoids have been absorbed into alcohol, the plant matter is strained and the tincture stored in an opaque dropper bottle.

Rick Simpson Oil (RSO)

Rick Simpson Oil is one of the most well-known forms of cannabis concentrate. Made popular by Rick Simpson, who cured his own skin cancer with cannabis. RSO is commonly used for medical purposes because of its extremely high potency.

RSO is made with solvents, though just about any solvent will do. Basically, RSO is a cannabis tincture that has been evaporated so much that only the black oil remains. However, due to the flammable nature of most solvents, the evaporation process can be very dangerous, especially if conducted over flame or direct heat, and is therefore recommended only for professional extraction.

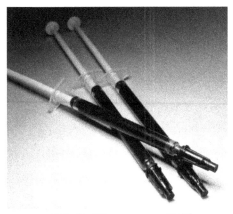

RSO is black like tar, which suggests that there is a high level of impurities in the oil, hence the birth of many modern cannabis extraction techniques that remove excess plant matter and other

Rick Simpson Oil

impurities. RSO is typically consumed orally or sublingually—under the tongue, although many who use it topically as well.

The Rick Simpson Story

Rick Simpson was an engineer working in 1997 in a Canadian hospital when he collapsed off of a ladder in the boiler room, becoming over-

whelmed by toxic fumes from the asbestos on pipes that were covered with potent aerosol glue and poor ventilation. In the fall, he hit his head and was knocked unconscious.

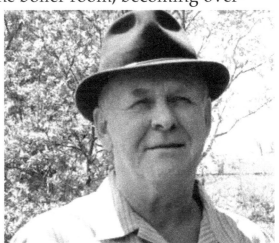

Rick Simpson cured his skin cancer with cannabis.

Simpson suffered from dizzy spells and a ringing in his ears for years after the accident, but his prescribed medication had little effect, even making his symptoms worse. After watching a documentary describing the positive benefits of using cannabis, Simpson began experimenting with medicinal marijuana. His tinnitus and other symptoms quickly showed significant improvement.

In 2003, three suspicious bumps appeared on Simpson's arm and were diagnosed as basal cell carcinoma, a form of skin cancer. Hearing about a study reported in the *Journal of the National Cancer Institute* in which THC was found to kill cancer cells in mice, Simpson wanted to use medicinal cannabis but was unable to find a doctor willing to help him. So Simpson decided to treat his skin cancer topically by applying concentrated cannabis oil to the cancerous spots, which he kept covered for several days.

After four days, when he removed the bandages, the cancerous growths were gone and Simpson became a true believer in the medicinal powers of cannabis. Through research and experimentation Simpson learned how to cultivate and harvest cannabis to create his own form of cannabis concentrate, now known as Rick Simpson Oil, or RSO.

Distributing cannabis oil to those in need became Simpson's mission, which he did free of charge—giving RSO to more than 5,000 cancer patients. Despite of his charitable work, Simpson faced persecution in his native Canada. His home has been raided the Royal Canadian Mounted Police and his plants confiscated on multiple occasions.

How Concentrates Are Used

Seasoned cannabis consumers often use concentrates to increase the intensity of their high, as well as to enjoy exquisite terpene tastes. Because concentrates are more efficient than flower, medicinal patients often use concentrates to achieve a direct, economical and fast-acting soothing of their ailments.

Cannabis concentrates are frequently called 'dabs' that come in many forms and are also referred to by numerous names such as kief, hash, CO_2 oil, butane hash oil (BHO), shatter, bubble hash, glass, wax, crumble, budder, rosin, nug run, and honey oil.

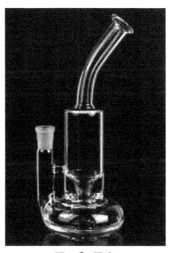

Dab Rig

Cannabis concentrates are consumed in a wide array of ways such as within tinctures, with a water bong or pipe, using a vaporizer or dab rig, cooked in edibles, or even rolled in a joint.

Cannabis concentrates are a great way to get really high really quickly, but many common methods of cannabinoid extraction have left out one of the most important parts of the plant: the terpene profile. Fortunately, evolving extraction methods are focusing on terpenes just as much as they are cannabinoids leaving us with more flavorful, more potent, and way more therapeutic cannabis concentrates.

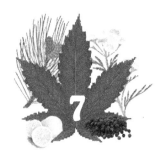

Consuming Terpenes

Terpenes are found throughout nature—not just in cannabis. Mother Nature has given us many ways to consume them. The more traditional ways of ingesting terpenes and the essential oils in which they are found include topical application, oral ingestion, diffusers, humidifiers, and perfumes applied to clothing, bedding, and skin.

While terpenes are readily absorbed through the nose, which is expected since they are so fragrant, terpenes are also absorbed through pores in the skin and in the salivatory glands of the mouth. Many essential oil and terpene distributors have created terpene-specific vaporizer pens designed to help calm the mind, stimulate creativity, and bust lethargy. When inhaled, special terpene blends can work instantly to reduce stress or invigorate the body, while their therapeutic potential is increased when consumed in conjunction with cannabinoids from the cannabis plant.

Consuming Terpenes With Cannabis

Because terpenes and cannabinoids are produced in the same part of the cannabis plant, consuming cannabinoids almost always includes the consumption of terpenes as well. Traditionally, this involves burning dried cannabis flower in a joint or pipe, then inhaling the smoke that comes from it, or by orally ingesting cannabinoids and terpenes in food or drink. However, terpenes evaporate at around 80 degrees Fahrenheit, so many burn up when smoking before they get into your body.

Smoking marijuana through a pipe or rolled up into a cigarette or "joint" is an easy way to enjoy the benefits of cannabinoids. However, to reap the full effect of terpenes, lower temperatures are required when baking with cannabis. Alternatively vaporized cannabis, which heats cannabinoids and terpenes only enough to evaporate them into the air but not so hot as to combust them into potentially carcinogenic—cancer-causing—substances making it a good method for consuming cannabinoids with terpenes.

Vaporizer Pens

Cannabis and cannabis concentrates can be vaporized by a few methods. There are a variety of vaporizer pens—vape pens—that can

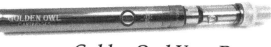

Golden Owl Vape Pen

be used for discrete, convenient cannabis and terpene consumption. The type of pen to use depends
on the level of terpenes to be consumed—versus
burned off. For example, those who want to experience the full flavor—and effects—of terpene-rich
cannabis concentrates should always use vape
pens with low or variable heat while those who
rather inhale large plumes of vapor and a deeper,
more pronounced sensation in the lungs are likely
to prefer higher temperature pens.

Types of Pens

Different types of pens are necessary for different
mediums. For example, vaporizer pens designed

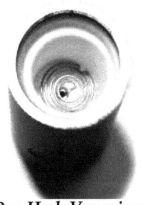

Dry Herb Vaporizer

to vape flower and dried
herbs rely on convection-style
heating in which a chamber
is heated to an even temperature using air circulation. Vaporizing herbs requires that
the chamber—the oven—to
be carefully packed so the air
can circulate easily while still
offering a warm, smoky "hit"
so many seek.

Wax-friendly vaporizer pens—which includes
concentrate types like wax, shatter, budder, rosin and live bubble hash—use heated wires at
the base of the chamber. The concentrate is best
vaporized when placed directly on the heating

elements. These types of vape pens regular up-keep is necessary to maintain proper functioning and require regular cleaning and replacement to maintain optimal performance.

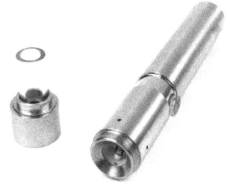

Wax Vaporizer

kingpenvapes.com

Vaporizor pens that work with pre-filled cartridges heat a coil at the base of the cartridge like wax vaporizers do, so there is less hassle of having to clean them often. Cartridges are usually single-use—although some are refillable—and are discarded when the cartridge runs dry but the battery can still be used. By comparison, because disposable pens do not separate the battery and cartridge, they must be completely replaced once the pen has run dry.

Note: many pre-filled cartridges use additional "thinning agents" to improve the consistency of concentrated cannabis. Some of the thinning agents used in cannabis concentrates include propylene glycol, vegetable glycerin, and medium chain triglycerides (MCTs), which have produced dangerous carcinogens like formaldehyde, acetaldehyde, and acrolein.

Researchers from the Medical Marijuana Research Institute in Tempe, Arizona, found propylene glycol produced the highest amount of formaldehyde and acetaldehyde byproducts of all the thinning agents that were tested, noting a significant increase in formaldehyde after heating the product to 450 degrees Fahrenheit. Both formaldehyde and acetaldehyde are cancer-causing carcinogens, suggesting that vaporizing products containing propylene glycol—a precursor to these carcinogens—may increase risk of developing cancer and other health complications.

Some thinning agents are safer for consumption. Cannabis concentrates produced with CO_2, for example, result in a thin, oily substance that is easily vaporized in standard vape pens making CO_2 extraction ideal for affordable, pre-filled cannabis vaporizer cartridges. However, traditional CO_2 extraction methods do not remove cuticle waxes—a thin layer of wax that forms on the surface of the plant—from their concentrates, which may build up in the lungs. The safest CO_2 extraction methods for vaporizer cartridges should therefore include the removal of these waxes through a winterization, which is an additional filtration process.

Perhaps the best thinning agent for cannabis concentrates are terpenes extracted from the cannabis plant or other natural sources, like mangos or blueberries. Terpenes are naturally very oily—

hence the abundance of essential oils donning the market. Terpenes can be extracted during the distillation process then reintroduced after all other impurities have been removed, making terpene-rich cannabis distillates a safe and pure way to consume cannabis concentrates, plus vaporizing rather than burning terpenes increases their therapeutic potential because they are not combusted.

Tabletop Vaporizers

Tabletop vaporizers are the original way to vaporize dried herbs and wax concentrates. The Volcano was the first tabletop vaporizer, made popular in the late 1990s as a healthier alternative to smoking cannabis. Tabletop vaporizers are popular in the medical community seeking a heavier "hit" of cannabinoids and larger plumes of vapor because a large dose of cannabinoids that can be consumed in a single sitting.

Tabletop vaporizers are heavier, larger, and more expensive than vaporizer pens. They come with a few additional

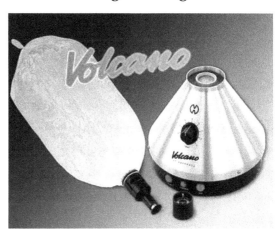

components and offer two different methods of inhalation—a long, hookah-like tube or a detachable, heat-resistant balloon. These two inhalation methods are beneficial for severely ill and disabled patients because they allow caretakers to prepare the vapor and pass it off to their patient as opposed to the patient having to take a "hit" directly from the apparatus.

Tabletop vaporizers use convection heating, which requires constant air flow to keep the temperature inside of the chamber where the cannabis flower or concentrates are loaded. Dried herbs, waxes and oils heat more evenly with convection heating and require lower temperatures to function properly, which is especially beneficial considering terpenes begin to vaporize at only 80 degrees Fahrenheit while cannabinoids don't begin to vaporize until 220 degrees Fahrenheit.

Convection-style heating allows for more even, accurate temperature control—which can be adjusted on the device itself depending on preference—making tabletop vaporizers ideal for both beginners and experienced consumers, but the cost of production—and thus the street price—tends to be higher than the conduction-style heating used in most hand-held vaporizer pens. Convection heating also takes longer to reach its optimal temperature, so patience is a must when using tabletop vaporizers.

Oil Pipes/Dab Rigs

Oil pipes, commonly referred to as "dab rigs" or "concentrate rigs", are special pipes designed for oil and wax inhalation. Home-based dab rigs often look like a water pipe or "bong", whereas portable dab rigs look like wands—called "nectar collectors". Both require the use of a heating element—either a blow torch or an electronic contraption called an electronic nail or an "e-nail".

A standard rig has four major parts: a mouth piece, a percolator that uses water to help filter carcinogens, a 90-degree joint, and a nail—literally looks like a nail or banger, which has a bowl shape that is better for hitting larger dabs. Arguably, the nail or banger is the most important component because this part that is heated and the piece on which the concentrate is placed for vaporizing. Domes and dab caps can also be used to reduce the amount of vapor that escapes into the air.

Oil rigs require a heating element—usually an electric heating element or, more traditionally, a

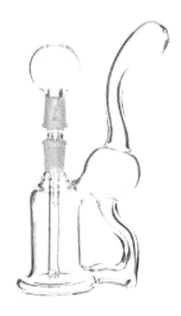

Pyrex Dab Rig

blow torch. When using a torch, extra time is required to heat the nail or banger to a glowing red color and patience is required to allow it to cool to an optimal temperature.

Low temperature "dabbing" takes place between 315 and 450 degrees Fahrenheit and is ideal for those who want a mellow experience with maximized flavor while minimal lung irritation. Medium temperature "dabbing" occurs between 450 and 600 degrees Fahrenheit and is used to achieve a more potent hit and deeper sensation in the lungs. However, such combustion causes development of dangerous carcinogens at the higher temperature range. High temperature dabs occur between 600 and 900 degrees—the temperature of the glowing-hot nail—and will be very harsh, will taste burnt, and will result in an extreme loss of cannabinoids and terpenes. Anything above 900 degrees will burn and should not be tried.

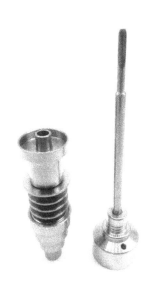

The process of heating a dab nail with a torch is complicated and potentially hazardous,

Dab with Titanium Nail

which is why electric nails are recommended instead. They plug into the wall or run on batteries and include a heating element that attaches to the nail or banger to heat the surface electronically. Electric nails allow for controlling the temperature of the device, though the material of the nail may cause variance in the actual temperature and quality of the dab. Titanium nails heat quicker and hold their temperature longer, for example, but the flavor tends to be poor with health concerns. By contrast, ceramic nails take longer to heat but are safer to use and tend to produce great flavor. The quality of a quartz nail depends largely on its thickness but tends to be a happy medium between the electric and titanium nails.

Combinations

Many people prefer flower but love the taste and potency of concentrates. Some may want a full terpene profile despite having less-than-flavorful flower—flower that has been poorly cured, for example, or old cannabis that's past its prime. In these cases, combining concentrates with flower—or adding additional terpenes to sub-par cannabis concentrates—can make a for a great cannabis experience.

The easiest way to combine different mediums is to simply "top"—add a small amount of concentrate to the top of a flower-filled bowl or pipe.

Topping improves the flavor of the flower as well as increasing its potency by helping it burn slower. Some may roll the wax between the hands into a kind of "log", which is put into a cannabis cigarette or by simply layering flower and concentrates in a pipe lasagna-style.

Another common method of combining different cannabis concentrates is the addition of supplemental terpenes to concentrated cannabis. Many distributors reintroduce terpenes into distilled cannabis concentrates. Home-based

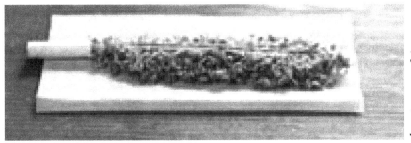

Wax oil rolled into log, then rolled into joint.

consumers can do the same effect by using dab rigs, tabletop vaporizers, or special wax-friendly vape pens, or by adding a terpene-rich concentrate like "terp sauce" to cannabis concentrates. Terp sauce is terpenes that have been extracted from a plant—generally a cannabis plant but not always—through a supercritical distillation process. The gooey, golden substance is simply concentrated terpenes that may or may not contain cannabinoids as well.

However, adding terpenes directly to the cannabis flower or concentrate is not needed to reap the dual benefits of each. In fact, many foods contain terpenes and consuming them, either before or after cannabis consumption, can alter the cannabis high that ensues. For example, mangos contain high levels of the terpene, myrcene, which increases the level of cannabinoids in one's system, increases the duration of cannabinoid presence in the blood, and speeds the onset of a cannabis high. Conversely, black pepper contains the terpene, beta-caryophyllene, which reduces the uncomfortable symptoms of cannabis overconsumption. Novice cannabis consumers may benefit by keeping a few peppercorns handy just in case their THC consumption gets the better of them.

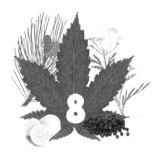

Flavonoids and Terpenes

There is a third class of chemicals in cannabis, besides cannabinoids and terpenes, with therapeutic potential—flavonoids. Flavonoids are the chemicals that provide pigment in plants—often yellows but they could be blues, reds, purples, or greens, as well—and appear most frequently in leaves and pedals to attract pollinators and deter pests. If you've ever wondered why some strains have such vivid colors—why the strain, Grape Ape, is always so purple, for example, the answer is because of flavonoids.

Flavonoids help protect plants from ultraviolet light by filtering out harsh rays. This is the reason sativa plants, which originated in the very sunny equatorial areas of

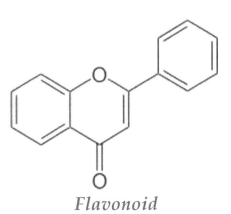

Flavonoid

the globe, tend to have deeper pigmentation—darker greens, reds and pur-ples—while indi-ca strains do not.

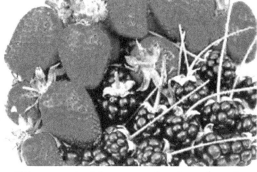

The pigmen-tation, especial-

Pigmentation protects plants.

ly blues and purples, help plants differentiate between various wavelengths of light thereby allowing the plant to respond to changing pho-toperiods. When the light cycle changes to lon-ger wavelengths—lights that appear to be red or orange—and shorter periods of light, cannabis plants receive the signal that summer is coming to an end and to finish their growth cycle by pro-ducing flowers or seeds for the next generation. This happens naturally during the months of Sep-tember and October in the United States but can be artificially simulated using special lights and timers in a grow room.

Flavonoids are not unique to cannabis, though. In fact, flavonoids are present in many fruits and vegetables as well as chocolate, tea and wine. Research suggests that foods rich in flavonoids help reduce the risk of cancers and cardiovascu-lar disease, which may explain why plant-based diets are so healthy.

Flavonoids, like terpenes and cannabinoids, are known to have amazing therapeutic potential as antioxidants, neuroprotectants, anti-inflammatories, and more. When consumed in conjunction with terpenes and cannabinoids, flavonoids contribute to the overall "synergistic effect" in which these chemicals work together to improve therapeutic benefit. Whereas THC alone has anti-inflammatory properties, for example, when taken alongside terpenes and flavonoids, the anti-inflammatory properties of each is heightened.

How Flavonoids Interact with the Body

Flavonoids interact with cannabinoid receptors in the body, much like terpenes and cannabinoids do, which may explain why they seem to have an effect on mood. Because cannabinoid receptors are pre-synaptic—occurring before electric signals are passed through the brain, they help control the way cells communicate with each other.

Though it was originally believed that flavonoids exerted their therapeutic potential exclusively through their antioxidant properties, recent research suggests that their interaction with the body may be more complex. According to a summary of flavonoids published by Oregon State University, "available evidence from cell culture experiments suggests that many of the effects of flavonoids, including anti-inflammatory, antidiabetic, anticancer, and neuroprotective activities, are related to their ability to modulate cell-signaling pathways." In other words, rather than simply cleaning up damage caused by the metabolic process and resulting free radicals, flavonoids directly affect the way cells send and receive signals. It is believed this allows them to induce cancer cell apoptosis, regulate insulin levels, and protect the brain from age-related degradation among other benefits.

Flavonoids "stick" to opioid receptors, which helps to regulate pain. Though most flavonoids bind weakly to opioid receptors, some flavonoids like cannaflavin—flavonoids found exclusively in cannabis—bond strongly enough to activate opioid signaling. In fact, research suggests that cannaflavin might actually work better than aspirin for pain management.

Some flavonoids, like green tea quercetin flavan-3-ol and genistein, may increase the toxicity of certain drugs when taken in conjunction. Though dietary intake of these flavonoids is generally considered safe, excessive intake may increase the toxicity of chemotherapeutic drugs, antifungal

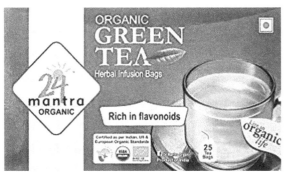

Green tea is rich in flavonoids.

agents, antihypertensive agents, HIV protease inhibitors, immunosuppressive agents, and some antibiotics. Always consult a physician to discuss drug interactions prior to beginning a flavonoid supplement regimen.

Classes of Flavonoids

More than 6,000 different flavonoids have been identified in nature, each of which can be categorized into one of six major classes based on its source and therapeutic potential.

Anthocyanidins: Anthocyanidins, which are red, blue and purple, can be found in berries, plums, pomegranates and red wine. Some of the specific flavonoids in this group include malvidin, pelargondin, peoidin and cyanidin and are known to promote heart health, reduce obesity, and prevent or control Type II diabetes in addition to their antioxidant properties.

Flavones: Flavones are a colorless crystalline that serve as the base for white and yellow pigments. They are found in celery, parsley and hot peppers, and benefit the body both with their antioxidant properties and their ability to slow the metabolism of certain drugs to help reduce the frequency in which they are consumed.

Flavanols: Falvanols, or flaven-3-ols, are a colorless chemical found in apples, teas, grapes, cocoa, and red wine and commonly contain catechins, which help lower cholesterol. Catechins may also reduce chronic fatigue and help improve cardiovascular and neurological health.

Flavonols: Flavonols—not to be confused with flav-a-nols—are commonly found in onions, broccli, beans, berries and tea. Flavonols include common flavonoids like quercetin, an antihistamine and anti-inflammatory, and kaempferol, an anti-inflammatory and antioxidant. Research suggests that flavonols found in cranberry juice may help prevent bacterial infection.

Flavanones: Flavanones make up the largest subgroup of flavonoids and are found in high concentrations in citrus fruits and mint. Flavanones are known to have a positive effect on cardiovascular health and cancer prevention and may improve bone health and reduce cholesterol. Pinocembrin, a flavanone found in honey, ginger, and oregano, may also have neuroprotective benefits as demonstrated in animal studies.

Isoflavones: Isoflavones are phytoestrogens or plant-based chemicals that act like the estrogen hormone in the body. As such, they may be beneficial in the treatment and prevention of hormone-related cancers like breast and prostate cancer. They may help reduce symptoms of menopause, though research on the subject is still too young to be conclusive. Isoflavones are found in high concentrations in soy products and legumes.

Flavonoids in Cannabis

There are 20 different flavonoids found in cannabis many of which—cannaflavins—are found exclusively in the cannabis plant, specifically in the leaves and stems, while none are found in the roots or seeds. Many of these flavonoids are soluble in water, which may explain why cannabis teas are seemingly so therapeutic despite the fact that cannabinoids are not water soluble—so the colors and flavors of the cannabis plant can be steeped into water, whereas cannabinoids like THC and CBD are not water-soluble.

Though research regarding cannaflavins has been limited due to legal restrictions of the controlled substance status of cannabis, what we know so far is pretty impressive. For example, cannaflavins A, B, and C inhibit inflammation by acting on the same pathway that cannabinoids and terpenes do suggesting that flavonoids, in conjunction with terpenes and cannabinoids, create an entourage effect of therapeutic benefits. Whereas

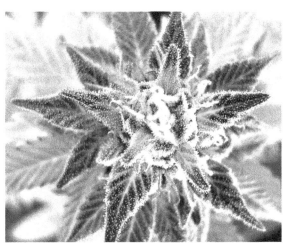

Flavonoids in cannabis

cannabinoids like THC and CBD exert strong anti-inflammatory properties, adding cannaflavins into the mix increases the potency of their anti-inflammatory actions.

Other cannaflavins like vitexin and isovitexin help regulate thyroid functions and improve gout symptoms while kaempferol has an antidepressant effect in addition to an anti-cancer and improved cardiovascular effect.

Apigenin, another cannaflavinoid, acts as an immunosuppressive, which may reduce the risk of transplant rejection in many patients. It is one of the few substances capable of altering neurotransmitter levels giving it anxiolytic—anti-anxiety—and sedative qualities.

Quercitin has anti-inflammatory and antiviral actions, but, unlike most other flavonoids, it can affect the rate at which neurotransmitters and some pharmaceutical drugs are metabolized. Consuming quercitin while using pharmaceuticals medicines should be done with caution because quercitin may increase the toxicity of pharmaceuticals drugs. Always discuss your proposed use with your doctor before using quercitin therapeutically.

Finally, luteonin and orientin are cannaflavinoids that protect the body against radiation thanks to their antioxidant properties, their ability to slow lipid metabolism and their ability to regulate immune system functioning. They are also able to protect healthy cells without interfering with programmed cell apoptosis, which suggests their long-time use could protect the body from cancers and gastrointestinal complications.

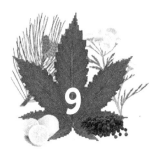

Cooking With Terpenes

Terpenes give cannabis—as well as many of our foods—their amazing flavor. Without terpenes, food would be bland and a marijuana "high" would be flat, with little taste. Given the importance of terpenes in both cannabis and foods, it makes sense that cannabis and food go so well together.

Professional chefs creating marijuana pairings, much like food and wine pairings, is one of the newest trends in fine restrauants, in which a chef carefully curates the perfect strain and food combination to bring out the flavor in both. Using terpene profiles to the pair of food and cannabis is popular. For example, the

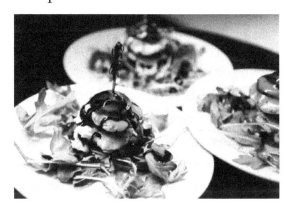

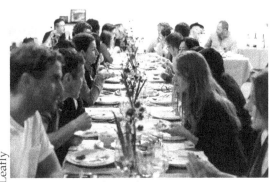

Leafly

Cannabis dinner party.

strain, Strawberry Cough, with its sweet, strawberry flavor, pairs well with a berry cobbler for a fruit smoothie. In high-end cannabis bistros, the dish could be infused with the strain while extra Strawberry Cough joint might be served on the side of the desert to smoke while enjoying the sweet treat.

Other common cannabis plus food pairings include the strain, Tangie, alongside citrus marinated salmon or lemon meringue pie because of the strain's strong citrus flavor, or the flavorful Agent Orange with a glass of Hefeweizen—a classic German wheat beer. Similarly, the cannabis strain OG Kush pairs well with barbeque or red meats because of its earthy, piney flavor.

The notion behind pairing strategies is that similar flavors accent each other. Consuming cannabis and food based on matching terpenes is an easy way to highlight the unique flavors of each while simultaneously showing off your cannabis expertise and impressing your friends.

Complementary Flavors

Alternatively, cannabis can be paired with food based on complementary terpenes instead of similar ones. Examples of this approach is pairing the sweet flavors of the strain, Blue Dream, with the bitter flavors of French onion soup or pairing the peppery flavor of the strain, Jack Herer with candied carrots. By choosing complementary flavors instead of matching ones, the subtleties of are easier to distinguish.

To pair cannabis with food based on the terpene profile, it's important to first understand the terpene profile of a given strain. The easiest way to do this is to ask a experienced budtender which strains are the most pungent. Then let your nose guide the way. If the strain smells sweet and fruity, pair it with something else sweet and

The human tongue can detect five types of flavors—sweet, salty, sour, bitter, and umami.

fruity or choose a dish that is not sweet, at all. The human tongue can detect five types of flavors—sweet, salty, sour, bitter, and umami. So food pairing can be based on whichever of these flavors and perfumes are detected from the cannabis flower.

Guides are available online to terpene profiles of various strains. However, much of cannabis's flavor and effects are subjective to one's personal taste buds. Flavor can vary from generation to

Umami means "savoriness" in Japanese. and can be experienced in foods such as mushrooms, anchovies, and mature cheeses, as well as in foods enhanced with monosodium glutamate, or MSG, a sodium salt derived from glutamic acid.

generation even within the same strain. Let your nose and taste buds determine which foods to pair with which cannabis strain.

There is no right or wrong way to pair cannabis and food. However, to avoid a bad experience with edibles: Start low—go slow to habituate to eating edibles.

Terpenes in High-End Edibles

Fewer people are consuming cannabis just to "get high" and are opting instead for a well-rounded experience. Though traditional methods for infusing cannabis into food simply involved mixing ground-up marijuana into a batch of brownies. Today, discerning consumers want more. While some edible producers initially turned their focus to trying to create infused treats minus the characteristic marijuana flavor, they quickly learned that consumers do, in fact, want to taste the cannabis they are eating—they just want it to taste good! Hence the newest trend in cannabis edible preparation: perserve terpenes..

The total amount of terpenes in cannabis edibles depends largely on the type of cannabis used to make the edibles. The traditional method of mixing dried marijuana into a pan of brownies included terpenes. However, the most volatile—and fragrant—terpenes evaporated out of the cured bud, leaving only the flavor of green plant matter behind.

Some edible manufacturers use distilled cannabis concentrates that do not contain any terpenes. This is a good method for those wanting to maintain the flavor of the food item itself while omitting the flavor of the cannabis, but it does little to address the synergistic qualities of using cannabinoids and terpenes together.

Professional chefs are making their way into the cannabis industry. Pulling from what we already know about the therapeutic benefits of terpenes, many edible cannabis companies are choosing particular strains to use based exclusively on their terpene profiles. For example, Periodic Edibles in Oregon has created a line of caramel candies infused with a lavender-flavored indica strain for a relaxing, end of the day treat.

Preserving the complete terpene profile in cannabis prior to edible infusion requires that the fresh cannabis

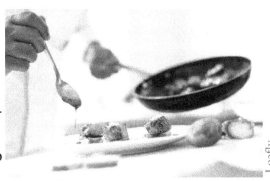

Cannabis chefs are creating new culinary experiences.

flowers, or "buds" be flash frozen prior to infusion. This keeps the terpenes from evaporating or otherwise degrading, which they commonly do during the curing process—the process of slowly drying cannabis flowers in preparation for later consumption. Though proper curing preserves many terpenes, the full profile can only be saved if the plant is frozen immediately after harvest. Otherwise, most terpenes quickly evaporate from the plant.

It's important to maintain low temperatures when infusing terpene-rich cannabis into food items. Many terpenes evaporate at temperatures as low as 80 degrees Fahrenheit so edibles containing terpenes should be both cooked and stored at low temperatures. Food items that must be cooked may have terpenes added after the edibles have drop below a certain temperature.

A Science

Terpenes are potent and extracts must be diluted before consumption. Adding terpenes to food is a science but not new. When adding a zest of lemon, for example, or a sprig of rosemary in cooking a meal, you are adding terpenes to food. Some of the most common terpene-rich foods include coriander, cinnamon, black pepper, cloves, as well as many other herbs and spices.

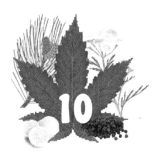

Pamper Yourself

Whether found in cannabis or in other natural sources, terpenes are powerful healing aids, capable of helping us live our healthiest—and most enjoyable—lives possible. Even better: you don't need to "smoke" anything or otherwise ingest them directly into your body. In fact, perhaps the most rewarding way to reap the benefit of terpenes is to purposefully pamper yourself with terpene therapeutics.

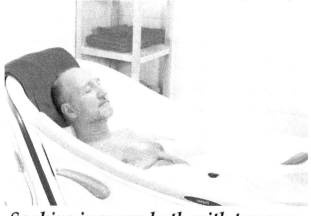

Soaking in warm bath with terpenes oils promotes well-being.

Using Terpenes In Your Bath

Though often overlooked, the importance of self-care should never be understated. One way to do so is to block out an hour or so each week to pause to enjoy the good things life available to you. A soak in the tub with a few favorite terpene oils is a great way to do just that. Soaking in a warm—not hot—bath provides much-needed alone time free from the distractions of the outside world, along with some great health benefits, as well.

Psychologist, Neil Morris from the University of Wolverhampton found that men who took warm baths every night for two weeks experienced a reduction in depression and pessimism. Morris attributed this to the nightly combina-

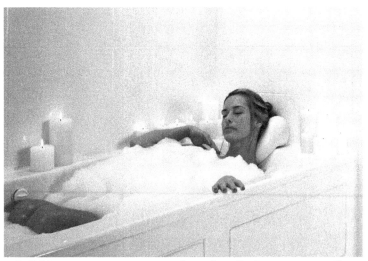

Adding terpenes to a hot bath increases the bath's therapeutic potential.

tion of isolation, quiet and comfort—much like being in a womb. Of course, it could also have something to do with a warm bath's ability to reduce muscle pain, reduce blood pressure, and induce production of the sleep hormone melatonin as the body's temperature drops after exiting a warm bath.

Adding terpenes to a hot bath increases the bath's therapeutic potential. Because terpenes evaporate at such relatively low temperatures, adding them to hot water helps them evaporate along with the water vapors so they can be absorbed through both the skin and the lungs. The water temperature of a hot bath should be between 100 and 104 degrees.

How to Add Terpenes to Your Bath

There are a few different ways you can use terpenes in a hot bath, the first of which is to simply add a few drops of your favorite terpenes to running bath water, which helps it mix thoroughly throughout the bath. Because terpene extracts tend to be so concentrated, only 15 milliliters—one tablespoon or roughly 12 drops—are necessary for a full standard-sized bath.

For added benefit, terpenes infused into bath salts are an excellent choice. Bath salts are made from Epsom salt—which is crystalized magnesium—and is often thought to help relieve muscle pain and com-

mon cold and flu symptoms. When infused with terpenes from the eucalyptus plant, Epsom salt can help
relieve muscle pain and congestion while Epsom salt
infused with terpenes from lavender can help relax
the body and melt stress.

Terpene Combinations

Lavender and Chamomile Oils:

Adding a combination of 10 drops of laven-

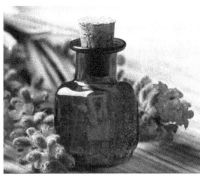

der and 5 drops of
chamomile oil to
your bath is a sooth-
ing way to end a
stressful day. Laven-
der is a sedative and
an antidepressant
while the chamo-
mile eases tension
and calms the mind.

Lavender is a sedative.

Frankincense, Lavender and Bergamot Oils:

When anxiety simply won't allow you to relax,
a combination of 10 drops frankincense plus
5 drops lavender plus 5 drops bergamot can
help. Frankincense relieves anxiety and often
brings about a contemplative mindset, while
bergamot reduces the production of the stress
hormone, cortisol, in lab rats. Lavender is
calming.

Rose, Frankincense and Coconut Oils Plus Sea Salt:

To transitioning from a hectic day at work to an invigorating evening on the town, equal parts of rose and frankincense—about 10 drops—plus coconut oil and sea salt in your bath can

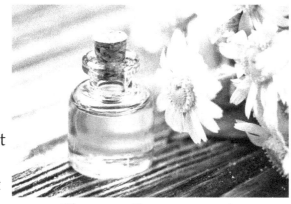

Chamomile eases tenion and calms the mind.

help. Rose oil will invigorate and uplift while the frankincense melts away work-related stressors. Adding coconut oil and sea salt increases absorption while helping reduce inflammation and other surface-level irritations.

Lavender, Citrus and Peppermint Plus Clove and Jojoba Oils:

Sore muscles don't stand a chance against this terpene combination of 10 drops lavender plus 5 drops of citrus and peppermint plus 1 to 2 drops of clove and jojoba oils. Whether caused by a strenuous workout at the gym or a tense day at work, using these oils in the bath will make those sore muscles relax again. Peppermint oil, cool against the skin, can increase blood flow to the muscles, cloves help numb the skin, and citrus helps rejuvenate from fatigue. Lavender with its ability to reduce tension is always a good addition.

Peppermint and Eucalyptus Oil:

The pain-relieving qualities of peppermint oil plus the decongestant properties of eucalyptus will stop a sinus headache. Just be careful not to splash; these terpenes are very powerful and can easily cause irritation to your eyes. Use 10 drops of pepperment and 5 drops of eucalyptus oils.

Rosemary, Lemon and Basil:

These oils—10 drops of rosemary plus 5 drops eahc of lemon and basil—are great for those days when you're feeling mentally fatigued. Whether you have a big project that's due soon

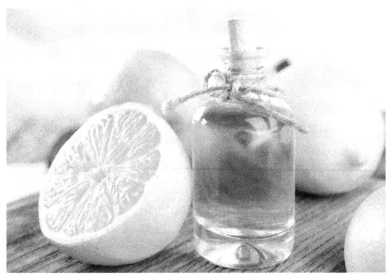

Lemon oil is mentally stimulating.

or you're trying to write the next best seller, sometimes you need a little mental stimulation to kick-start your intellectual engine. To do this, just add these essential oils to a running bath and soak for 30-45 minutes. Lemon oil is mentally stimulating while rosemary is known for helping promote memory retention. Basil helps stimulate the mind and to inspire creative thinking.

Clary Sage Plus Chamomile and Lavender:

Feminine issues like menopause or PMS can leave the body feeling fatigued, bloated, irritable and in pain. Using 5 drops of clary sage oil in your bath can reduce these symptoms by stimulating estrogen production combined with 2 to 3 drops of lavender and chamomile oil work to relieve tension and irritability.

CLARY SAGE

Terpene Topicals

When a 30-to-45-minute bath simply isn't an option, adding terpenes directly to the skin can be a quick alternative.

Clary sage can reduce bloating.

However, because essential oils are so concentrated, they should always be diluted prior to application. While lotions and other topical creams are ready

to use topically, mixing a few drops into coconut oil is often enough. Though some essential
oils are safe to use without diluting them—rose,
lavender, and chamomile, for example, diluting
essential oils is always recommended for use with
children and seniors, as well as else when you're
unsure of their potency.

Do not add terpenes to areas of the body that
are especially sensitive, including the eyes or
genitals, as this can cause irritation. Having said
that, essential oil application can occur just about
anywhere else—behind the ear, on wrists or feet,
or even directly on the problematic area—like
temples in the case of a headache. Never rub essential oils into broken skin and discontinue use
if irritation occurs.

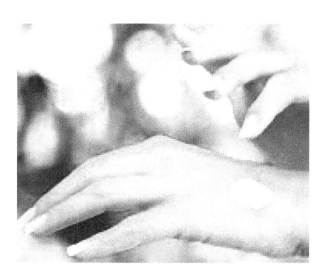

*Topical
creams
are easy
to use.*

Terpene Diffusers

Aromatic terpene diffusers are helpful when topical application or lengthy baths are not an option. They combine the steamy benefits of a warm bath with the convenience of bed-side—or table-side—relief. Diffusers come in many styles and add to ambiance—and therapeutically beneficial terpenes—to any room. Whether using one

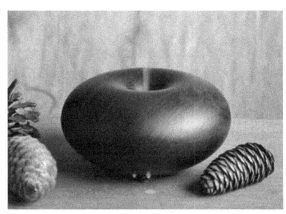

Ultrasonic diffuser.

that's low-profile or one that serves as an attractive centerpiece, terpene or essential oil diffusers are a wonderful gentle way to reap the benefits of terpenes in the air.

When choosing a diffuser, avoid those that require heat as it can disturb the delicate chemistry of the terpenes. Steam diffusers, candle diffusers and hotplates are examples of diffusers to avoid.

Of course, there are many diffusers that do not require heat to work, the most popular of which being ultrasonic diffusers, which work by vibrating quickly to break down the essential oils into tiny particles that disperse into the air as a fine mist. Conversely, nebulizing diffusers produce a stronger scent by vaporizing the terpenes before dispersing them into the air. These tend to be more expensive than ultrasonic diffusers, and tend to be more difficult to clean.

Outdoor Terpenes

Earlier we discussed the benefits of forest bathing—spending time in forested areas—to improve health by inhaling the surrounding natural terpenes. Because of the dense plant growth in forested areas, natural terpenes are abundant, taking a hike in the woods is especially beneficial. Thusly, by consciously spending time in nature, focusing closely on the therapeutic ingestion of vital terpenes, you can improve your health and longevity while developing strong, healthy habits.

One way to do this—aside from taking a daily walk in the woods—is to practice yoga in a terpene-rich environment. There are many benefits to practicing yoga regardless of age including increased flexibility, improved blood flow, weight management, balanced metabolism, and protection from injury. Additionally, yoga encourages you to focus on breathing patterns, which helps oxygenate the blood to help reduce toxins and increase energy. When practicing mindful breathing through yoga, you can increase the rate at which terpenes enter the body to improve health and healing.

Terpenes may also improve cardiovascular health and increase endurance. By exercising in terpene-rich environments, you can strengthen your heart and increase stamina to keep blood flowing and muscles moving effortlessly.

The most terpene-dense environments are those with a lot of vegetation. If you cannot get to a forested area easily, a city-funded botanical garden or even a private garden area filled with fragrant vegetation will do wonders for your spirit and your body.

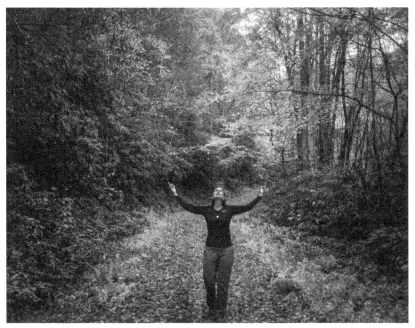

The forest is filled with natural terpenes.

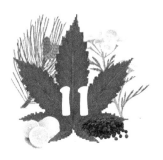

Terpenes in Herbal Teas

Another enjoyable way to ingest terpenes is in herbal beverages like teas and other plant-infused drinks. There are only four "true" types of teas: oolong, black, green, and white tea, all of which are actually different preparations of the plant, *camellia sinensis*. However, herbal beverages such as those made from flowers, herbs and spices, are commonly referred to as teas, as well. Herbal beverages may also be called herbal infusions, botanical infusions, or tisane to reduce confusion with true teas. For the sake of

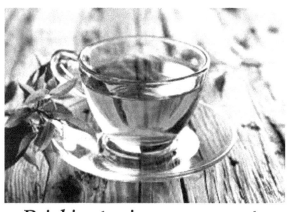

Drinking tea is an easy way to consume terpenes.

discussion, we will refer to them interchangeably as both herbal teas and herbal beverages.

Herbal beverages are made by steeping dried flowers, fruits, leaves, stems and roots of various plants in hot water, which can improve the antioxidant status, and reduce oxidative stress in humans, especially when consumed in conjunction with a healthy diet. Some herbal beverages such as those made with citrus, ginger, and rosehips are also good for pregnant and breastfeeding mothers while others like oregano, peppermint and thyme are best avoided when pregnant.

Herbal beverages, complete with their full myriad of terpenes, flavonoids, alkaloids and more, can have a profound effect on bodily functioning. Some may

Some teas have powerful antioxidant, antibacterial, antiviral, anti-inflammatory, antiallergic qualities.

reduce breast milk production while others show powerful antioxidant, antibacterial, antiviral, anti-inflammatory, antiallergic qualities. Some herbal beverages, especially true tea beverages, may also help regulate metabolism and aid in weight loss.

While there are hundreds of herbal plants and plant combinations that are used to make herbal infusions, following is a list of common herbal beverages along with a brief summary about what they do to treat the body so well.

Chamomile Tea

In addition to its anti-inflammatory and antibacterial properties, chamomile tea is a great way to promote a good night's sleep. One study found that those who consumed chamomile extracts twice daily were more likely to sleep throughout the night compared to placebo. Another study found chamomile to reduce symptoms of depression and improved quality of sleep. Chamomile may also help ease stomach discomfort and stabilize blood glucose, insulin and lipid levels.

Chamomile tea for a good nights sleep.

Peppermint Tea

Though peppermint can block bacteria, viruses, oxidation, and possibly retard some cancers from forming in the body, it's most commonly used to treat stomach issues like indigestion, nausea and stomach pain, and may also reduce spasms along the digestive tract. Nine different studies analyzing 726 patients found peppermint oil can significantly reduce symptoms of irritable bowel syndrome and reduce abdominal pain as compared to placebo suggesting that peppermint oil may safely and effectively treat IBS for a short time.

Peppermint tea eases tommy problems.

Ginger Tea

Ginger-infused beverages have long been known for their ability to ease nausea, especially as it relates to pregnancy, motion sickness, and cancer treatments. It may also help ease the discomforts of constipation and indigestion and works as well as ibuprofen at relieving mild pain and body aches. Studies also suggest that ginger may help improve diabetic symptoms by regulating blood sugar and lipid levels.

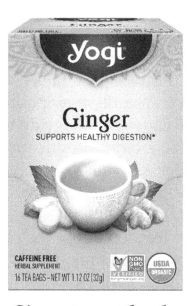

Ginger tea settles the stomach.

Rooibos Tea

Rooibos is a South African red bush that has been used as a medicinal tea for centuries. Though evidence regarding its effectiveness at treating allergies and kidney stones is inconclusive, research suggests that rooibos tea can help stimulate the cells responsible for bone growth and density. Researchers believe it is the plant's ability to reduce inflammation and cell toxicity which may be why drinking rooibos tea is associated with higher bone density.

Rooibos tea   Additionally, rooibos tea
strengthens bones may improve heart health by
and improves   inhibiting the production of
                     the enzyme that causes blood
vessels to constrict. One study found that drinking
six cups of rooibos tea each day for six weeks low-
ered "bad" cholesterol and increased the production of "good" cholesterol.

Cannabis Tea

Consuming cannabis leaves and stems in tea is a
wonderfully therapeutic way to enjoy the flavors
of cannabis alongside therapeutic terpenes and
flavonoids without any risk of getting "high".
That's because cannabinoids, like THC, are not
water-soluable. Cannabinoids are soluable in
fat or alcohol, but not water, in which they can-
be leached out of the plant. Unless cannabis is
steeped in milk, which has fat, or infused into a
tincture with an alcohol base, the chances of any
cannabinoids making their way from a tea into
the blood—and brain—are slim.

For those who prefer a bit of a body buzz, cannabis tea can be made on the stovetop with milk,
cream, or some other fatty liquid. Cannabis stems
work well in these cases, but a larger quantity is
required as the cannabinoid level in stems is very
low. Nevertheless, terpenes in the stems are plen-
tiful and easily absorbed into water for a relaxing,
flavorful way to reap the benefits of therapeutic
terpenes in the cannabis plant.

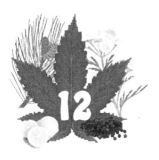

Terpene Toxicity

Terpenes act within the body in profound ways. They are often used to benefit health through their wide range of therapeutic applications, but this does not mean they're beneficial to everyone all the time. Some concentrated terpenes, such as those found in essential oils, can be toxic when used improperly, especially when used around young children and older adults. To ensure that everyone in the household remains as happy and healthy as possible, exercise caution when handling terpenes and essential oils.

Terpene Sensitivities

Terpenes can irritate the skin and lungs if used improperly. Children under the age of two and seniors are especially prone to irritations caused by terpenes and essential oils so it's important to

Some concentrated terpenes can be toxic when used improperly.

practice safe handling when used around them. This includes proper dilution—more so for those with sensitive skin—and minimal topical use until there are no allergic concerns.

Some photosensitive oils, or oils that react to ultraviolet rays, can pose a threat to sensitive skin. Even those without sensitive skin who do not properly dilute oils prior to topical application may be burned when exposed to the sun or tanning beds for an extended length of time. Citrus-based terpenes are especially phototoxic—i.e., dangerous when exposed to light on the skin—and can cause burns and increase risks of skin cancers. Lotions and essential oils containing these terpenes should always be thoroughly diluted and monitored closely in case a rash occurs.

Certain terpenes should not be used topically in the sun, others should not be used topically at all, especially for people with sensitive skin. Cinnamon, cloves and lemongrass oils, for example, should not be used on sensitive skin as they are well-known to cause irritation. Fortunately, irritation is usually localized at the site of application and can be remedied by washing the area with soap or bathing in a fatty milk bath of two percent or higher, according to the American College of Health and Sciences.

Inhaling Terpenes

Inhaling terpenes is the safest and most efficient way to ingest valuable terpenes, but there are special considerations to take into account when doing so. For example, while diffusion is the easiest way to inhale terpenes at home, it should always be done in a well-ventilated area and never for more than 30 minutes at a time. It's also important to follow dilution instructions

Inhaling terpenes is the safest and most efficient way to ingest them.

precisely and to always ensure that pets—especially cats—can leave the room if their experience is overwhelming. Importantly, pets tend to be more sensitive to the effects of terpenes so always exercise caution when pets are present.

Some terpenes, such as those found in eucalyptus or peppermint oils, can be beneficial in treating short-term respiratory problems—when you're suffering from a head cold, for example—but may damage the airways if used for a prolonged amount of time. Children and seniors are especially prone to bronchial discomfort after inhaling these terpenes as are pregnant women who can easily transport terpenes to the fetus through the placental barrier. Some rare oils are also known to cause miscarriage. So pregnant women should be especially cautious.

Over-use of some essential oils can cause an allergy, as well. Whereas an individual may react fine to a new oil, frequent use can cause the body to develop a sensitivity to it. A toxic reaction to essential oils containing a specific terpene may cause the individual to experience adverse reactions to the naturally-sourced terpene, as well.

Such was the case for Rachael Armstrong from Omaha, Nebraska, who experienced rashes and severe burning after regularly lathering herself with bergamot and lemon oils. The blisters healed, and rashes cleared up with the use of steroids but to this day, her aversion to lemons continues. Even freshly sliced lemon will cause Armstrong to break out in hives, likely because her body is trying to defend her from another toxic occurrence.

What To Do If a Reaction Occurs

Many people are under the false impression that natural means safe. While Mother Nature has been known to deliver powerful therapeutic plants, like cannabis or other terpene sources, allergic reactions are common. Poison oak is "natural" but look what happens if you touch it! Two people rarely react to the same substances in the exact same way so individual tolerance and sensitivity should be monitored closely.

The first sign of terpene toxicity is usually the appearance of a red, itchy rash. Formally called Allergic Contact Dermatitis, this rash usually occurs at the site of the

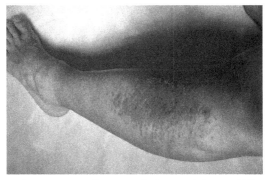

Some with sensitive skin will develop a rash.

application though it could be present throughout the body if the oil was taken orally. The rash should clear up after ceasing use, provided that it is the source of the rash in the first place. Remember that an allergic reaction does not always occur after the first application. Just because a rash didn't occur the first time does not mean it won't cause a rash later.

A skin rash following the use of essential oils could be caused by an allergic reaction to plant pollens in the oil and not the terpene itself. To help determine the source of the allergic reaction, switch brands then try a small, diluted sample on the skin at the fold of the elbow twice daily for three to five days. If a reaction occurs, the allergen is the terpene, if the reaction subsides, it's likely due to an impure oil.

Unlike Allergic Contact Dermatitis, Contact Urticaria is an allergic reaction that happens immediately, much like a bee sting. This type of allergic reaction can cause difficulty breathing; swollen lips, tongue and throat; a drop in blood pressure and hives. These reactions to essential oils are rare and have yet to be fatal, but consumers should be aware, no less.

To reduce the chances of an allergic reaction to terpene oils, never use the same combination of terpenes for more than a few months; always test new oils on a small patch of skin inside the elbow, and use extra diluted oils around children, seniors, and pregnant women.

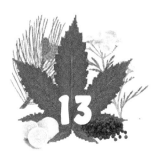

Terpenes and Pets

Many terpenes that are safe for humans are not safe for pets, even in very small doses. Whereas environmental terpenes are typically considered safe around pets, terpene oils—essential oils—are very potent and can cause toxicity in small animals. For example, using or diffusing essential oils in small, poorly-ventilated areas may pose a threat to household pets, especially cats and birds because of their sensitive respiratory systems. The ASPCA advises against all essential oil diffusion around birds because of their sensitive respiratory systems and recommends avoiding specific oils around other pets, as well.

Terpenes are potent and can cause toxicity in small animals.

Additionally, topically-applied terpenes can cause irritation to a pet's sensitive skin. Though pet hair usually protects their skin from this in the wild, when terpene oils come into contact with the skin, it can easily absorb into the bloodstream causing liver damage and irritations to the skin surface. If a pet licks the oil off its skin or fur, it can cause gastrointestinal problems like irritation, nausea, diarrhea, and so on. If untreated, these issues can lead to long-term complications like liver failure, paralysis, or even death.

Dogs have very sensitive olfactory receptors.

Finally, remember that dogs, in particular, have very sensitive olfactory receptors. While a small dose of terpenes may be relaxing to you, too much may cause stress and exacerbate health problems in the canine population. The best way to avoid this issue is to use diffusers away from pets or to at least give them the opportunity to leave the room if the odor becomes uncomfortable for them. Do not use terpene oils directly on any pet's skin or fur and always monitor your pets closely for signs of distress.

"Natural" Doesn't Mean "Safe"

Pets are part of the family, and many pet parents want to treat their fury babies to the best foods and pet supplies their money can buy. Savvy marketers know this and often use this information to sell products based on buzz words that the general population seems to flock to: "organic" and "all natural", for example. But just because a product is labeled as "natural" or "organic" does not necessarily mean it's safe for your pets. Again, poison oak is "natural" but it is certainly not good for your skin!

Because of the relatively low toxicity levels of most terpenes and essential oils, the Environmental Protection Agency considers their use to be safe with minimal risk. This means the use of terpenes and essential oils is not tightly regulated. Pet supplies like shampoos, flea and tick collars and other pest treatment options may employ the use of terpenes or essential oils and be marketed without full disclosure of the possible risks involved. Specifically, some terpenes that can protect against pests may be dangerous to the very pets they're intended for.

Of particular concern are pet shampoos that include limonene, or citrus to kill ticks and fleas. Because citrus-based terpenes tend to be very photosensitive, their use on sensitive pet skin can cause burning or other painful irritations. Linalool is also used to kill ticks and fleas on pets but can absorb into the bloodstream through the skin causing stomach discomfort like nausea, diarrhea and vomiting, and can cause liver damage and even death in severe cases. Other popular terpenes used in pet shampoos and flea collars that should be avoided include tea tree oil, geranium oil, bay oil, lavender and eucalyptus. Always monitor your pet closely when starting any new regimen and consult your veterinarian if any concerns arise. Report any rashes or localized irritations immediately to avoid infection.

Terpenes to Avoid Around Pets

Dogs, cats, and birds all process terpenes differently. Signs of an adverse terpene reactions also vary by species so it's important to understand which terpenes your pets can tolerate as well as potential toxic reactions to them.

Dogs

A dog's adverse reaction to terpenes is usually in the form of skin sensitivities and allergies. However, because dogs tend to lick irritated spots on their skin, the likelihood of them ingesting a dangerous amount of terpenes increases when there is an allergic reaction to them.

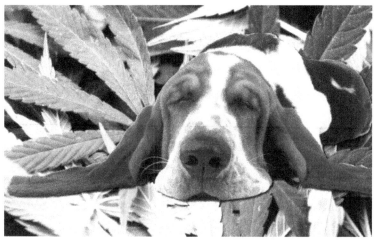

thuglifevideos.com

The most common oils that fall in this category include horseradish, juniper, cloves, cinnamon, pine, sweet birch, thyme, wintergreen, anise and yarrow. If your dog ingests a toxic amount of terpenes from these oils, it may become weak or groggy, have difficulty breathing or walking, vomit, paw at its face and mouth, experience muscle tremors or break out in a rash of small red bumps—if eaten, the rash would be around its mouth and tongue. If your pet's breath or fur smells strongly of essential oils, likely it got into some. Monitor closely and treat quickly.

If you suspect your dog has gotten into essential oils, do not induce vomiting as this could make the condition worse. Instead, take the suspected essential oil with you to your veterinarian immediately so they can treat your pup safely. If the oil is on the skin or fur, wash the area immediately with mild soap like dishwashing detergent.

Cats

The use of essential oils is much more complicated around cats. Their bodies lack a special enzyme that makes it difficult to process and expel many essential oils. This can lead to a toxic build-up of certain essential oils compounds, especially those containing phenols and phenolic compounds—that are responsible for the "flavor" of many essential oils unlike terpenes which are responsible for the "odor" of essential oils.

These compounds are extremely corrosive and can cause burns that penetrate many layers of the skin, inhalation can cause severe respiratory issues while ingestion—either orally or through the skin—can cause liver failure. Birds and reptiles are also sensitive to phenolic compounds in essential oils. Some examples of essential oils that contain polyphenolic compounds include cloves, oregano, thyme, tea tree, cinnamon, birch, and wintergreen.

Monoterpenes terpenes are also toxic to cats and include oils like terpineol, limonene and pinene. Because of their extreme sensitivity to these compounds, the list of oils to avoid around cats is quite extensive.

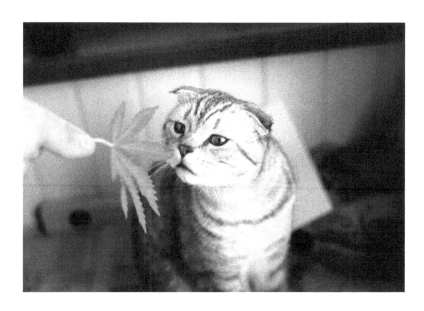

Below is a list of terpenes to avoid around your cat along with treatment options should an allergic or toxic reaction occur.

Keep These Terpenes

Away From Cats

Bergamot	Frankincense	Pine
Birch	Grapefruit	Rue
Bitter almond	Horseradish	Sassafras
Calamus	Juniper	Savory
Camphor	Lavender	Spearmint
Cassia	Lemon	Spruce
Citronella	Lemongrass	Tangerine
Cinnamon	Lime	Tansy
Clove	Mandarin	Tea Tree
Coriander	Mustard	Thyme
Cypress	Orange	Verbena
Eucalyptus	Oregano	Wintergreen
Fir	Peppermint	

Symptoms of essential oil toxicity in cats include drooling, tremors, vomiting, instability, low blood pressure and respiratory distress. If any of these symptoms are present, or if you smell essential oils on your cat, seek immediate veterinary assistance. Don't forget to take all packaging

with you to your visit along with a detailed time-
line outlining consumption and symptom details.

Using Terpene Oils Safely Around Pets

Just because you have pets doesn't mean you can't
use terpene-based essential oils. Though there
certainly is a long list of oils to avoid, some essential oils can be used around pets as long as they are
thoroughly diluted and not applied directly to the
skin. It is also recommended that you keep all essential oils out of paw's reach and to never diffuse
essential oils in poorly ventilated areas.

When dealing with cats, birds, reptiles or rodents, avoid air diffusers all together—even in
well-ventilated areas—and keep pets out of any
rooms that require them. Keep the bathroom locked
if you're adding tea tree or eucalyptus oils to a bath,
for exam-
ple. Finally,
remember to
monitor all
household
pets closely
when essen-
tial oils are used—or even present—in the home.
If you notice a shortness of breath, watery eyes,
unexplained lethargy or an inability to move easily,
consult your veterinarian immediately.

When dealing with cats, birds, reptiles or rodents, best to avoid air diffusers all together—even in well-ventilated areas.

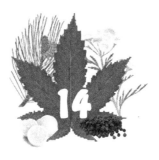

Terpenes and Seniors

As our bodies age, maintaining a healthy lifestyle can become a challenge. It's vital to remain active—both physically and mentally, eat healthy, and surround ourselves with positive people and situations if we are to live the longest lives possible. One helpful way for seniors to maintain a healthy routine is by incorporating terpenes and terpene oils into their daily regimen.

Different terpenes provide various therapeutic benefits. Interestingly, we tend to be drawn to the specific terpenes our bodies need. Perhaps this is the reason certain terpene scents appeal to us more than others. Linalool from lavender flowers, for example, may appeal to someone whose body needs a good rest while limonene from citrus fruits may be more appealing to those needing to focus or maintain productivity. Whether at a

> *We tend to be drawn to the specific terpenes our bodies need.*

dispensary or grocery store, pay close attention to the smells you are drawn to then figure out a way to get the related terpenes into your routine to improve your personal wellness.

Because the world of terpenes is so vast, determining the specific terpenes your body craves can be a challenge until you become more familiar with the characteristics and therapeutic benefits of several popular terpenes. Therefore, in this chapter we will discuss how specific terpenes can help maintain wellness, especially for seniors or baby boomers who tend to experience a multitude of health problems concurrently. Terpene therapy can be especially beneficial for seniors when used as part of a regular daily routine. Below is a list of some of the most common senior ailments along with which terpenes and flavonoids to use to help treat them

Terpenes for Anxiety and Depression

Until recently, it was believed that anxiety and depression diminish as we get older. However, recent research suggests that seniors experience anxiety and depression at the same rate as the younger population—it's just reported less often. According to the *International Journal of Geriatric Psychiatry*, around 27 percent of seniors show signs of anxiety, which may reduce their interest ability to perform regular daily tasks. Reduced socialization, inability to move without pain, or sheer frustration at the increasing difficulty of performing daily tasks can exacerbate feelings of anxiety and depres-

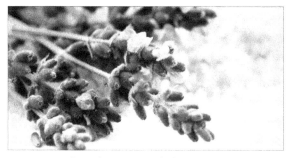

Linalool is good for soothing anxiety and depression.

sion among seniors, which may also reduce their quality of life and lifespan in general.

Linalool is one of the best terpenes for treating anxiety and depression. One mouse study found that even small amounts of linalool can reduce aggressive tendencies and increase socialization. Beta caryophyllene, a common terpene found in herbs like rosemary, hops, and black pepper, has also been shown to reduce the symptoms of depression and anxiety in animal models.

Terpenes for Inflammation

Inflammation is the most common cause of pain, especially among seniors. Commonly caused by arthritis—which is basically a swelling at the joints that may be caused by a thinning of cartridge or by the body attacking the lining of the joints. Inflammation can make it difficult to bend, sit, walk, or move. When someone experiences chronic inflammation such as with arthritis, their

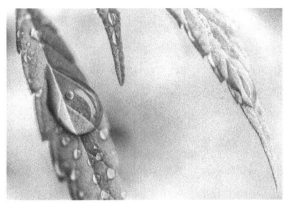

Myrcene in cannabis relieves joint inflammation.

mobility and their overall satisfaction with life can dwindle, as well.

Though the most common methods for treating arthritis include regular rest and exercise, the pain caused by the inflammation can make these simple tasks difficult to accomplish. Fortunately, many terpenes can reduce joint inflammation such as myrcene, the most prominent terpene found in cannabis. Alpha-pinene can also reduce inflammation in the joints while beta-caryophyllene helps reduce inflammation along the gastrointestinal tract.

Terpenes for Gallstones

Gallstones are the most common gallbladder problem among seniors. They are formed from bile, cholesterol and calcium deposits and can become lodged in bile ducts causing acute pain in many individuals. Women are especially prone to gallstones, especially senior women who experience rapid weight loss or gain, or those with a family history of gallstones.

Though *Menthol, pinene, borneol, camphene,* 80 percent *cineol and menthone are terpenes* of people *that, when used in conjunction with* experience *a healthy diet rich in fiber, can help* no adverse *dissolve gallstones.* symptoms of gallstones—which often pass on their own— some may become lodged in the body causing pain and inflammation. Because many medications do not effectively break down gallstones, surgery may be recommended. Unfortunately for the senior population, surgery carries an additional set of complications because the body cannot always heal efficiently after invasive procedures.

Seniors who experience painful gallstones may fair better by incorporating specific terpenes and flavonoids into their diets. Menthol, pinene, borneol, camphene, cineol and menthone are just a few terpenes that, when used in conjunction with a healthy diet rich in fiber, can help dissolve gallstones.

Terpenes for Glaucoma

Glaucoma is a cluster of diseases that is characterized by excessive pressure in the eyeballs. Glaucoma is most common in seniors over the age of 60, especially those of Mexican or African descent. It is a genetic disorder characterized by malfunctions to the optic nerve and can cause irreversible vision loss if not treated.

Fortunately, eye pressure caused by glaucoma can be mediated with the use of a few simple terpenes and flavonoids. Specifically, terpenes from grape seed and pine bark can help treat and prevent chronic glaucoma as can flavonoids from blue and red berries.

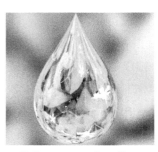

Myrcene is the most sedating terpene in cannabis.

Terpenes for Sleep

The ideal amount of sleep a person should get every day does not decline with age. Unfortunately, many seniors have an increased diffculty falling asleep and staying asleep, which can lead to more health-related complications down the road. Unfortunately, many common senior ailments like pain and depression can block ability to get a restful night's sleep making it more difficult for the body to repair itself after injury or illness.

Fortunately, many terpenes have been shown to promote sleep, with or without the inclusion of cannabinoids like THC. Myrcene is perhaps the most sedating terpene in cannabis—known for causing the couch-lock effect—while linalool may help reduce the symptoms of depression and anxiety that keep people awake at night. In small doses, pinene can help slow the mind to promote longer sleep cycles though high concentrations can have the opposite effect.

Bibilography

--------- 3 Common and Dangerous Essential Oil Mistakes. American College of Healthcare Sciences. (n.d.), Aug 15, 2017.

Alchimia, The Entourage Effect: Synergy between cannabinoids and terpenes. *Alchimia Blog: News About Marijuana and Growing Guide*, 2018, May 04.

American Association for Clinical Chemistry (AACC). "Any dose of alcohol combined with cannabis significantly increases levels of THC in blood." *Science-Daily*, 27 May 2015.

_____ Anxiety in Older Adults, *Mental Health America*, April 28, 2015.

ASPCA, Is the Latest Home Trend Harmful to Your Pets? What You Need to Know!, *ASPCA News*, January 17, 2018.

Barrett, M.L., D. Gordon, and F. J. Evans, Isolation from cannabis sativa L. of cannflavin—a novel inhibitor of prostaglandin production, *Biochemical Pharmacology*, V. 34, # 11, 1 June 1985, pg 2019-2024.

Beckman, A., Coffee and Cholesterol – Is There Cause for Concern? Choleslo-Review.com, *Cholesterol Management Information and Advice*.

Booth, J. K., Jonathan E, Page, Jorg Bohlmann. Terpene Synthases From Cannabis Sativa, *PLoS One*. 2017; 12(3): e0173911. Björn Hamberger, Editor

Can Baser, K. H., & Buchbauer, editors. *The Handbook of Essential Oils; Science, Technology and Applications*. CRC Press, 2010.

Chandrasekara, Anoma and Fereidoon Shahidi Herbal beverages: Bioactive compounds and their role in disease risk reduction - A review. Vol. 8, no. 4, October 2018, pg 451-458.

——Code of Federal Regulations Title 21. (CFR). Food and Drugs: Chapter I-Food for Human Consumption, Part 182.20 , Substances Generally Recognized as Safe.

Chang, S. M., & Chen, C. H. Effects of an intervention with drinking chamomile tea on sleep quality and depression in sleep disturbed postnatal women: A randomized controlled trial. *J. Advanced Nursing*, 2016 Feb, 72(2):306-15.

Cho, K. S., Lim, Y., Lee, K., Lee, J., Lee, J. H., & Lee, I., Terpenes from Forests and Human Health. *Toxicological Research*, 2017, Apr., Vol. 33(2), pg 97-101.

Elisabetsky, Elaine. Ethnomedicine and Drug Discovery, *Advances in Phytomedicine,* 2002

Gertsch, Jürg, Marco Leonti, Stefan Raduner, Ildiko Racz, Jian-Zhong Chen, Xiang-Qun Xie, Karl-Heinz Altmann, Meliha Karsak, and Andreas Zimmer. Beta-caryophyllene is a dietary cannabinoid. *PNAS, Proceedings of the Academy of Sciences of the United States of America*, July 1, 2008 105 (26) 9099-9104.

Goodman, Brenda. Even Mild Anxiety May Shorten a Person's Life. *WEBMD*, July 31, 2012.

Gordon, B. In hot water? Have a bath and relax. Bryony Gordon on the healing and restorative power of taking a bath. Telegraph Media Group, 14 Oct 2002.

Guenther, E. *The Essential Oils – Vol II.* 456 pg., Ulan Press, 2012

HU, Frank B., Plant-based foods and prevention of cardiovascular disease: an overview, *The American Journal of Clinical Nutrition*, Vol. 78, No. 3, 1 September 2003, pg 544S–551S.

Janero, D. R., & Makriyannis, A. Terpenes and Lipids of the Endocannabinoid and Transient-Receptor-Potential-Channel Biosignaling Systems, *ACS Chem Neurosci.* 2014 Nov 19; 5(11): 1097–1106.

Kathy. Natural Flea and Tick Treatments That Are Dangerous to Dogs. *Creating a NewSense,* April 2015.

Khanna, R., MacDonald, J. K., & Levesque, B. G. Peppermint oil for the treatment of irritable bowel syndrome: A systematic review and meta-analysis. *J Clinical Gastroenterol.* 2014 Jul. 48(6):505-12.

Kobayashi, M., Wakayama, Y., Li, Q., Inagaki, H., Katsumata, M., Hirata, Y., . . . Miyazaki, Y. (n.d.). Effect of Phytoncide from Trees on Human Natural Killer Cell Function. *International Journal of Immunopathology and Pharmacology*, Oct., 2009.

Labuda, I., & Burns, F. J. Methods of blocking ultraviolet radiation and promoting skin growth using terpenes and terpenoids. US Patent Application: US20110158921A1, 2011, pending 2014.

Lancaster, J., Ashot Khrimian, Sharon Young, Bryan Lehner, Katrin Luck, Anna Wallingford, Saikat Kumar B. Ghosh, Philipp Zerbe, Andrew Muchlinski, Paul E. Marek, Michael E. Sparks, James G. Tokuhisa, Claus Tittiger, Tobias G. Köllner, Donald C. Weber, Dawn E. Gundersen-Rindal, Thomas P. Kuhar, and Dorothea Tholl. De novo formation of an aggregation pheromone precursor by an isoprenyl diphosphate synthase-related terpene synthase in the harlequin bug. *PNAS: Proceedings of the National Academy of Science of the United States of America*, 2018, September 11.

Levich, Nick and Tommy Joyce, *Key to Cannabis Blog*, Low Temp Dabs vs High: The Perfect Temperature for Dab Potency and Flavor.

Linck, V. M., Da, A. L., Figueiró, M., Caramão, E. B., Moreno, P. R., & Elisabetsky, E., Effects of inhaled Linalool in anxiety, social interaction and aggressive behavior in mice. *Phytomedicine.* July 17, 2010.

Link, Rachael, The 6 Best Teas to Lose Weight and Belly Fat. *Healthline Red.* Sept 25, 2017.

Linus Pauling Institute, Flavonoids, Oregon State University, https://lpi.oregonstate.edu/mic/dietary-factors/phytochemicals/flavonoids. Sept, 2018.

Marshall, L. Essential Oils: Natural Doesn't Mean Risk-Free. *WEBMD Health News,* Aug 8, 2017.

McKernan, K. Microbes and Terpenes. *Medicinal Genomics* Jan 2017.

Nash, L. A., & Ward, W. E. Comparison of black, green and rooibos tea on osteoblast activity. *Food Function,* 2016 Feb. 7(2):1166-75.

Persson, I. A., Persson, K., Hägg, S., & Andersson, R. G. (2010, May). Effects of green tea, black tea and Rooibos tea on angiotensin-converting enzyme and nitric oxide in healthy volunteers. *Public Health Nutrition,* 2010 May 13(5):730-7.

Rao, Suresh, Manjeshwar Shrinath Baliga, Polyphenols in the Prevention and Treatment of Vascular and Cardiac Disease, and Cancer**,** *Polyphenols in Human Health and Disease, 2014.*

Schmidt, B. M., & Cheng, D. M.. *Ethnobotany: A phytochemical perspective.* Hoboken: Wiley-Blackwell. 2018.

Souza-Alves, João Pedro, Natasha M. Albuquerque, Luana Vinhas, Thayane S. Cardoso, Raone Beltrão-Mendes, and Leandro Jerusalinsky. Self-Anointing Behaviour in Captive Titi Monkeys. *Primate Biol.,* 5, 1–5, 2018.

Stela Gilanová, Stela. Sztómás betegek életminőség-vizs-
gálata Szlovákiában, *Acta Medicinae Et Sociologica,*
2016, 7(22-23), 48-79.

Troutt, W. D., & M. D. DiDonato. (2017, November).
Carbonyl Compounds Produced by Vaporizing
Cannabis Oil Thinning Agents. *J. Alternative Comple-
ment Med.,* 2017 Nov. 23(11):879-884. doi: 10.1089/
acm.2016.0337.

Twohig-Bennett, C., & Jones, A. The health benefits of the
great outdoors: A systematic review and meta-analysis of greenspace exposure and health outcomes.
Environmental Research, Vol. 166, October 2018, pg
628-63.

Worcester Polytechnic Institute, Study shows cranberry
juice is better than extracts at fighting bacterial infections, Oct 28, 2011.

Yamada, Yuuki, Tomohisa Kuzuyama, Mamoru Komatsu,
Kazuo Shin-ya, Satoshi Omura, David E. Cane, and
Haruo Ikeda. Terpene Synthases Are Widely Distributed in Bacteria. *PNAS: Proceedings of the National Academy of Sciences of the United States of America,*
2014, Dec 22.

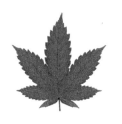

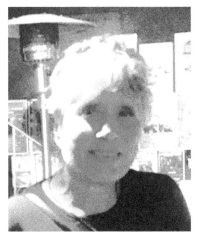

Docpotter

Beverly A. Potter, PhD ("Docpotter") earned her doctorate in counseling psychology from Stanford University and her masters in vocational rehabilitation counseling from San Francisco State University. She is a corporate trainer, public speaker and has authored numerous books on health and workplace issues like overcoming job burnout, managing yourself for excellence, high performance goal setting, mediating conflict, healing magic of cannabis, marijuana recipies (as Mary Jane Stawell), drug testing for employers and passing the test for employees.

Docpotter is based in Oakland, California. Her website—docpotter.com—is packed with useful information. Please visit.

Abby Hauck is a cannabis writer and founder of Cannabis Content, a marketplace designed to help cannabis enthusiasts become writers in the industry.

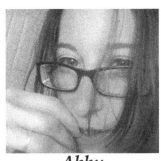

Abby

Other Books by Docpotter

The Healing Magic of Cannabis
It's the High that Heals!

Marijuana Recipies & Remedies for Healthy Living
as Mary Jane Stawell

Cannabis for Seniors

Cannabis for Canines

Overcoming Job Burnout:
How To Renew Enthusiasm For Work

Finding A Path With A Heart:
How To Go From Burnout To Bliss

The Worrywart's Companion:
21 Ways to Soothe Yourself & Worry Smart

From Conflict To Cooperation:
How To Mediate A Dispute

Get Peak Performance Every Day:
How to Manage Like a Coach

High Performance Goal Setting:
Using Intuition to Conceive & Achieve Your Dreams

Brain Boosters:
Foods & Drugs That Make You Smarter

Drug Testing At Work:
A Guide For Employers And Employees

Pass the Test: An Employee Guide to Drug Testing

The Way Of The Ronin:
Riding The Waves Of Change At Work

Turning Around:
Keys To Motivation And Productivity

Preventing Job Burnout: A Workbook

Youth Extension A-Z

Beyond Consciousness:
What Happens After Death

Patriots Handbook

Spiritual Secrets for Playing the Game of Life

Simple Pleasures

Question Authority to Think for Yourself

Managing Yourself for Excellence
How to Become a Can-Do Person

Healing Hormones
How to Turn On Natural Chemicals to Reduce Stress

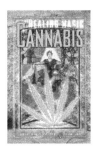
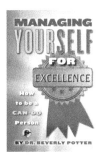
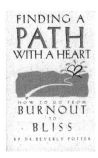
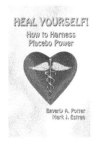
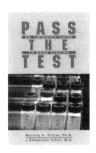
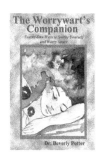
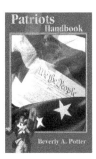
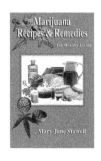
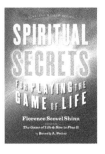
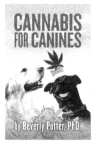
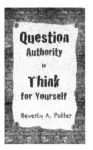
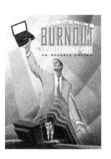
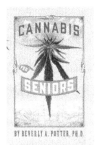
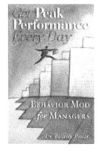

Printed in the USA
CPSIA information can be obtained
at www.ICGtesting.com
JSHW012013140824
68134JS00024B/2387

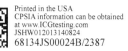

9 781579 512729